SUPPORTIVE CARE
OF THE
SURGICAL PATIENT

SUPPORTIVE CARE
OF THE
SURGICAL PATIENT

William M. Stahl, M.D.

Professor of Surgery,
New York University School of Medicine,
New York

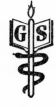

Grune & Stratton

NEW YORK AND LONDON

Library of Congress Cataloging in Publication Data

Stahl, William M.
  Supportive care of the surgical patient.

  Includes bibliographical references.
  1. Therapeutics, Surgical. I. Title.
[DNLM: 1. Postoperative care. 2. Preoperative
care. W0 178 S781s 1972]
RD51.S8   617'.91   72-8778
ISBN 0-8089-0786-7

Grune & Stratton, Inc.
111 Fifth Avenue
New York, New York 10003

Library of Congress Catalog Card Number 72-8778
International Standard Book Number 0-8089-0786-7
Printed in the United States of America

Do not Therefore imagine, that from this Time your Studies are to cease; so far from it, you are to be considered as but just entering upon Them; and unless your whole Lives are one continued Series of Application and Improvement, you will fall short of your Duty.

Samuel Bard, "A Discourse Upon the Duties of a Physician," Commencement, King's College, New York, May 16, 1769

CONTENTS

PART III.   Regulatory Systems

7.   LIVER   **189**

ACKNOWLEDGMENT

I wish to thank those who worked with me in the development and preparation of the manuscript: Emily Falk as editorial assistant, Ann Jefferson as secretary, and Howard Goldman as medical student reader and critic. Their assistance was most valuable.

W. M. S.

INTRODUCTION

Surgery is that portion of the healing art which treats the patient by physical means, usually incision, excision, or repair. For thousands of years this art was practiced as a simple mechanical endeavor, the results depending on the plastic skills of the operator and the unknown ability of the body to heal. It is only in the past half-century that an understanding of normal bodily function has been gained. Starting with this knowledge the response of the human organism to injury has become a matter for discussion and investigation [1, 2].

Works of Cannon [3, 4], Selye [5], and Moore [6] have provided guidelines for an understanding of the mechanisms which normally maintain the body in a state of health and which respond to restore this state when alterations are imposed. An understanding of these survival mechanisms is increasingly a concern of the surgeon.

Surgical judgment and technical expertise are major contributions which the surgeon can make to ease his patient's problem. If the survival systems of the individual are sufficiently strong and well-regulated, the outcome will be successful. Frequently, however, these systems are damaged, sluggish, or inoperative, and the surgeon's knowledge must be broad enough to provide proper physiologic and emotional support until the patient can regulate his own body economy satisfactorily. This book is concerned with the optimizing of these survival systems.

HOW DOES MAN SURVIVE?

The evolution of the unicellular organism into a complicated being of many billions of cells required specialization to a high degree. Sys-

1

tems were developed for the intake of energy substances and the disposal of metabolic products, for the transport of materials throughout the body, and for the regulation of the internal milieu. One may approach this complex organism by analyzing those mechanisms that regulate exchange with the environment, those that provide transport mechanisms from the exchanging area to the interior of the body cells, and those concerned with the maintenance of neural, chemical, and emotional stability.

ENVIRONMENTAL EXCHANGE MECHANISMS

The intake of certain elements and expulsion of others to achieve a balance within the organism takes place through four basic systems.

The respiratory system provides for gas exchange, allowing intake of oxygen and release of carbon dioxide (CO_2) and carbonic acid (H_2CO_3). The alimentary tract provides for uptake of energy substrates and evacuation of nonmetabolized wastes. The kidneys excrete the nitrogen resulting from protein metabolism, and regulate water, solute, and fixed acid concentrations. The skin functions as a protective layer to conserve water and to regulate body heat exchange.

TRANSPORT MECHANISMS

The transport systems of the body consist of the cardiovascular system, providing gross transport of vital substances to tissue beds, and the body fluids, within which microtransport of ions occurs.

REGULATORY MECHANISMS

The maintenance of a satisfactory internal milieu is accomplished by a variety of regulatory mechanisms. The liver, because of the many metabolic functions of liver cells, acts as a regulatory organ. The endocrine glands contribute to the regulation of all the exchange systems and are primarily concerned with the interstitial, membrane, and intracellular aspects of transport and metabolism. The operation of the autonomic nervous system contributes to regulation of all the exchange systems and to the functioning of the cardiovascular aspects of the transport system.

EMOTIONAL FACTORS

The emotional state of the individual plays an important role in the overall response of his survival systems. Certain emotional states such as fear and anxiety clearly affect the endocrine and autonomic nervous systems. Other less obvious emotional states may also alter the functioning of vital systems.

DISEASE

It is clear that the classification of body systems into exchange, transport, and regulatory mechanisms emphasizes one aspect of each system. While this aspect may be seen as a primary role, a complex interaction of all systems is needed for proper function of the body. As Claude Bernard stated, "All the vital mechanisms, however varied they may be, have only one object, that of preserving constant the conditions of life in the internal environment." [7]

A state of disease may be said to exist when these exchange, transport, and maintenance systems function at less than optimal levels. Such alterations may be due to a variety of causes ranging from congenital abnormalities to the degenerative changes of aging. In the early years of life the congenital phenomena may be of great importance, whereas in patients past middle age the changes due to degenerative processes, trauma, and previous infection most frequently hamper adequate response of vital systems.

INJURY

Trauma, whether accidental or surgical, may interfere with normal function in a variety of ways. The concept of a "metabolic response to injury" is a documentation of the alterations in normal exchange, transport, and maintenance mechanisms precipitated by a physical assault on the intact organism. Patients may present with chronic defects in survival systems, to which these acute changes are added. Secondary or indirect chemical and metabolic alterations often provide the final blow to the functioning of vital systems.

PLAN OF THE BOOK

In the following pages each of these survival systems having to do with envirionmental exchange, internal transport, maintenance of milieu, and emotional mechanisms will be discussed. For each system a review of the basic concepts of function will be presented, and the measurement techniques useful in assessing the adequacy of the system will be outlined.

Proper preoperative evaluation of the patient should provide the physician with clues to malfunction of vital systems. Adequate preoperative preparation of the patient requires assessment of likely deficits and correction of these as far as possible. Optimal intraoperative care requires support of vital systems through the physiologic disturbances imposed by anesthesia and operation. Proper postoperative management depends on the detection of early signs of failure of supportive systems, prevention of further deterioration, and correction of deficits as they appear. The maintenance of optimal function of vital systems constitutes the supportive care of the surgical patient.

REFERENCES

1. Moore, F. D.: Clinical surgery and biological science. Ann. Surg. 158:785, 1963.
2. Dragstedt, L. R., and Clarke, J. S.: The contributions of physiology to surgery, 1905–1955. Int. Abs. Surg. 100:205, 1955.
3. Cannon, W. B.: The wisdom of the body. New York, Norton, 1939.
4. Cannon, W. B.: Bodily changes in pain, hunger, fear, and rage. New York, Appleton, 1915.
5. Selye, H.: The general adaptation syndrome and the diseases of adaptation. J. Clin. Endocrinol. 6:117, 1946.
6. Moore, F. D., and Ball, M. R.: The metabolic response to surgery. Springfield, Ill., Thomas, 1952.
7. Bernard, C.: Leçons sur les Phénomènes de la vie Commune aux Animaux et aux Végétaux. Paris, Baillière, 1878.

PART I

Exchange Systems

I

RESPIRATORY SYSTEM

PRIMARY FUNCTION

The respiratory system provides the mechanism for exchange of gaseous elements between the individual and the surrounding air. This exchange is accomplished by exposing flowing blood to inhaled gas across the semipermeable alveolar membrane. Owing to differential partial pressures of specific gases, exchange occurs between alveolar air and blood. The utilization of oxygen by body cells during metabolic activity requires that oxygen be continuously exchanged from alveolar air into the circulation for delivery to the body-cell mass. Carbon dioxide produced by cellular metabolism must effectively be moved from the blood into the alveolar air.

The primary function of the respiratory system—the exchange of oxygen and carbon dioxide between blood and air—must be carried out continuously at a rate appropriate for the level of metabolism; otherwise rapid and destructive changes will occur. Oxygen tensions in circulating blood and in tissue fall rapidly if respiration is deficient. The maximum oxygen content of the blood at any moment can support life for only 10 to 15 minutes.

Carbon dioxide as a dissolved gas in the blood is a weak acid. Unless it is continuously removed from the blood into the alveolar air the level of blood acid (H^+ ion) rises precipitously. The excretion of H^+ ion approximates 15,000 mEq (milliequivalents)/24 hr. Cessation of respiration, therefore, results in the very rapid accumulation of carbonic acid in the blood with the production of respiratory acidosis.

7

ANATOMY

The human respiratory appratus is structurally designed to allow the exposure of a maximum amount of gas to a maximum amount of blood at any given time. It also provides for inflow and outflow of gas in order to bring fresh alveolar content into apposition with blood. It allows adequate blood flow through the alveolar capillary bed. The actual respiratory zone occupies approximately 90 per cent of the total volume of the respiratory apparatus, with the conducting airways and vessels making up the remaining 10 per cent. Of the respiratory zone, the alveoli occupy 57 per cent, the air ducts 27 per cent, and tissue and smaller blood vessels 6 per cent. These values apply in young individuals. Gradual changes occur with aging. In older individuals the alveolar fraction is reduced to 52 per cent, with the duct fraction increasing to 32 per cent [1-1].

Alveoli

Anatomic studies have found that all lungs, regardless of the size of the individual or his age, contain an equal number of alveoli (about 300 million), and alveolar ducts and sacs (about 14 million). The alveolus appears to be somewhat similar in shape to the cell of a honeycomb and is approximately spherical. The mean diameter of the alveolus ranges from 250 to 290 microns (μ), and the total exchanging surface of all the alveolar tissue ranges from 40 to 80 square meters (sq m), increasing with the size of the lung.

Capillaries

A network of alveolar capillaries surrounds each alveolus in a hexagonal mesh, with the total capillary surface similar in extent to the total alveolar surface. Seen under electron microscopy, the interalveolar septa measure approximately 100 millimicrons ($m\mu$) in thickness [1-2]. They are made up of endothelial cells, a small amount of mucopolysaccharide interstitial substance, and the lining epithelial cells of the alveoli.

Conducting Airways and Vessels

On the average, the conducting airways reaching to the 300 million alveoli have 23 generations of dichotomous branching, while the pulmonary arteries reach the 280 billion capillary segments after approximately 28 generations. In both the airway and the vascular systems the average diameters seem to be in agreement with the principle of minimum resistance and minimum mass.

The mucous membrane of the tracheobronchial tree is made of ciliated epithelium with frequent mucous-producing glands. The walls contain elastic fibers and circular smooth-muscle fibers. Cartilages are present down to the bronchioles of approximately 1 mm in diameter.

FUNCTIONAL REQUIREMENTS

Adequate functioning of the respiratory system depends upon (1) adequate oxygen content of the inspired gas, (2) an open-airway conducting system, (3) adequate area of functioning alveolar membrane, (4) apposition of this membrane to an adequate number of functioning pulmonary capillaries, (5) ventilation of alveoli sufficient to continuously provide adequate partial pressure of oxygen and to remove carbon dioxide, and (6) adequate flow of blood (cardiac output) through pulmonary capillaries.

Control of Respiration

A stimulus which acts to maintain adequate ventilation in man is anoxemia, measured by a fall in P_aO_2.* Increased minute ventilation occurs when the P_aO_2 falls below 60–70 mm Hg. This reflex is mediated by chemoreceptors in the aorta and carotid arteries. Increase in P_aCO_2 is a strong mechanism for increasing ventilation and is sensed in the medullary respiratory center. The aortic and carotid oxygen sensors are resistant to drugs and anesthesia, whereas the CO_2 sensor in the medulla is readily depressed by anything which depresses brain function. De-

* The terminology for expressing gas pressures uses lowercase letters for liquids in which gases are dissolved, as P_aO (partial pressure of oxygen dissolved in arterial blood) and P_vCO_2 (partial pressure of carbon dioxide dissolved in venous blood). Capital letters signify gas-phase pressures, as PAO_2 (partial pressure of oxygen in alveolar gas).

crease in blood pH due to an increase in metabolic acid content is also a stimulus to increase in respiratory minute volume. This increase acts to return the pH toward normal by producing compensatory respiratory alkalosis.

Pulmonary stretch reflexes (Hering-Breuer) also are present. These reflexes respond to overinflation or underinflation of the lung, thus regulating depth of tidal volume and so influencing respiratory rate. They arise within the pulmonary parenchyma and are mediated by the vagus nerves. They consist of two types. The *inflation* or *inhibito-inspiratory* reflex checks inspiration when the lungs have been inflated to a certain volume or degree of stretch. The *deflation* or *excito-inspiratory* reflex causes earlier and more rapid inspiration and acceleration of respiratory rate, triggered by deflation or collapse of portions of the lungs. Stimulation of these reflexes may occur in conditions where alteration in the pulmonary parenchyma is present. A possible example of this is the hyperventilation syndrome with resulting alkalosis seen in traumatized or septic patients.

Content of Inspired Gas

Air contains 80 per cent nitrogen and 20 per cent oxygen. At sea level, atmospheric pressure measures 760 mm Hg, of which approximately 47 mm Hg is produced by water vapor. Of the remaining pressure, oxygen represents approximately 159 mm Hg. Variations in inspired oxygen content from 20 to 100 per cent may be achieved by appropriate mixture of pure oxygen and air. One hundred per cent oxygen can provide approximately 673 mm Hg partial pressure of oxygen. These values will change at altitudes above or below sea level. High altitudes, with lower atmospheric pressure, provide less partial pressure of oxygen. At 15,000 ft the barometric pressure is 445 mm Hg, and the average P_aO_2 is 50 mm Hg. Higher atmospheric pressure than that at sea level can be obtained by the use of a hyperbaric chamber, the usual limit being 3 atmospheres of pressure and the obtained airway oxygen pressures ranging near 2000 mm Hg.

Arterial Oxygen

Adequate airway oxygen levels are needed to produce the required level of dissolved oxygen within the circulating pulmonary capillary blood. Arterialized blood issuing from the pulmonary capillary bed must contain a partial pressure of oxygen of at least 60–70 mm Hg to produce a saturation of hemoglobin approximating 90 per cent and to provide adequate oxygen transport at reasonable cardiac output levels. Oxygen is transported as dissolved gas and as oxyhemoglobin in erythrocytes. Transport as oxyhemoglobin is by far the most important mode. Dissolved oxygen at P_aO_2 of 95 mm Hg measures only 0.29 ml/100 ml whole blood, and a fall in P_aO_2 to 40 mm Hg, as occurs in passage through the capillary bed, contributes only 0.17 ml/100 ml whole blood to cellular metabolism. Oxyhemoglobin, on the other hand, at 97 per cent saturation, carries 20 ml/100 ml whole blood and contributes 4.6 ml/100 ml whole blood to cellular metabolism, as saturation falls to the venous level of 75 per cent. Oxyhemoglobin transport thus accounts for 96 per cent of oxygen delivery. Similarly, CO_2 transport is mainly achieved by transport of combined rather than dissolved CO_2, 95 per cent of CO_2 usually being in the combined form. Partial pressures of oxygen above 100–110 mm Hg produce very little increase in oxygen content of the blood, since hemoglobin is already 100 per cent saturated. A fall in partial pressure of oxygen below 60 mm Hg causes a rapid decrease in saturation of hemoglobin and triggers an increase in respiratory effort.

REGULATION OF ARTERIAL OXYGEN

The therapeutic concept of titration of airway oxygen concentration by mixing pure oxygen and air is physiologically sound and is monitored by measurement of P_aO_2. The object is to maintain the P_aO_2 between 70 and 100 mm Hg. The danger of prolonged use of airway oxygen concentrations higher than 70 per cent has been emphasized. Although the exact mechanisms are not yet known, it is safer to use the lowest oxygen concentration in the inspired gas that will produce the desired P_aO_2. Many of the commercial respirators indicate per cent oxygen concentration with certain dial settings. These may not be entirely accurate. Airway oxygen should be measured by an oxygen-sampling device.

Ventilation: Total and Alveolar

Ventilation (V), the movement of respiratory gas in and out of the lungs, must be maintained at an adequate level to provide constant alveolar gas exchange. This exposes the alveolar membrane to adequate oxygen levels and reduces the carbon dioxide tension of alveolar air to that of the inspired gas. Ventilation is described by the term *ventilatory minute volume,* which is the amount of air moved in and out of the respiratory apparatus per minute, $(\dot{V})$. Alveolar ventilation per minute $(\dot{V}_A)$ is that portion of the respiratory minute volume which reaches functional alveolar membrane. $\dot{V}_A$ is equal to the ventilatory minute volume minus the volume of nonexchanging pulmonary dead-space (V_D). V_D is the volume of the air passages extending from the intake area for fresh gas down to the alveolar duct, plus the volume of any alveoli not in contact with functioning capillaries. Tidal volume (V_T) is the volume moved in and out of the respiratory apparatus with each breadth.

PATTERN OF VENTILATION

It is quite clear not only that total ventilation or respiratory minute volume must be adequate, but that the pattern of respiration should be appropriate to maintain minute alveolar ventilation at an adequate level. Thus rapid shallow respirations with a tidal volume of 300 ml and a respiratory rate of 40 would produce a respiratory minute volume of 12 liters. If the dead-space measures 150 ml, then minute alveolar ventilation, which is the functional portion of the total minute volume, would measure 6 liters of the 12 liters total. By contrast, a tidal volume of 600 ml and a respiratory rate of 20 would produce a similar respiratory minute volume of 12 liters/min. With the same dead-space of 150 ml, the alveolar ventilation would rise to 9 liters of the 12 liters total, an increase in efficiency of 50 per cent.

OXYGEN CONSUMPTION

Oxygen consumption by the individual is regulated by the level of metabolism. For each level of oxygen consumption there is a level of alveolar minute ventilation required to provide gas exchange. For reference, a 75-kg male has an average oxygen consumption of 250 ml/min and needs approximately 4.3 liters/min of alveolar ventilation.

TISSUE HYPOXIA

It is vitally important to maintain a P_aO_2 of at least 60 to 70 mm Hg. If P_aO_2 and related arterial saturation fall much below this level, tissue anoxia occurs. Tissue vascular beds become dilated owing to local release of vasodilator substances or to relaxation of anoxic smooth muscle or both, and cardiac output rises in an attempt to increase oxygen delivery by increasing the flow of the circulation. The ability to maintain a hyperdynamic circulation may be limited in disease states and failure of cardiac function to maintain the elevated level leads to cell hypoxia, acidosis, and death.

HYPERVENTILATION AND HYPOCAPNIA

Decrease in the P_aCO_2 due to hyperventilation produces a decrease in blood flow to the brain by a reflex mechanism. This may be significant enough to cause mental changes in elderly patients who may already have limited cerebral blood flow due to atherosclerosis. Marked decrease P_aCO_2 can cause dizziness and mental clouding, even in normal individuals. It is possible for hyperventilation due to a P_aO_2 below 60 to 70 mm Hg to be associated with low P_aCO_2 levels because of the rapid diffusion of CO_2 across the alveolar-capillary membrane. Carbon dioxide diffuses 20 times as fast as oxygen.

Hyperventilation in the presence of P_aO_2 values above 60 to 70 mm Hg is occasionally seen in association with the posttraumatic and septic state, and may be the first indication of the development of the pulmonary insufficiency syndrome associated with these conditions.

HYPOVENTILATION AND HYPERCAPNIA

Elevation of the P_aCO_2 indicates hypoventilation. This elevation is never due to pure diffusion block and is almost never due to pulmonary shunting unless the shunt is greater than 50 per cent of the cardiac output. Thus an elevation in P_aCO_2 is indicative of widespread lung destruction as seen in severe emphysema or pulmonary fibrosis or, in the absence of severe chronic lung disease, to decrease in pulmonary alveolar ventilation [1-3]. It is an indication for clearing of the airway, mechanical assistance to ventilation and, if persistent, to tracheostomy. A markedly elevated P_aCO_2 can affect the brain with progressive mental clouding leading to unconsciousness. Acidosis produced by CO_2 retention may produce serious cardiac arrhythmia, especially when combined with hypoxemia, as is usually the case.

WORK OF BREATHING

The work of breathing is the effort expended in moving air in and out of the respiratory apparatus. Normally an optimal combination of tidal volume and respiratory rate exists to provide the alveolar ventilation required by the metabolic rate.

With slow deep respirations, air-flow resistance is minimized because flow is more laminar in nature and less turbulent. Work against elastic lung elements and chest wall is increased, however. Rapid shallow respirations produce more turbulent flow and greater airway resistance, while work against structural elements is decreased. In the usual situation the optimum balance is the midpoint of moderate air-flow rate and moderate tidal volume. Alterations in airway diameter due to stenoses or spasm, or changes in compliance, may shift this optimal point.

This balance is especially important in older individuals because of changes in pulmonary function due to aging. Anatomically, bronchial structures occupy a larger part of the respiratory tissue in elderly people, with resultant increase in dead space. Also, the work of breathing is increased due to increased resistance to air flow and changes in elasticity of the lung and chest wall [1-4].

Pulmonary Circulation

Adequate alveolar ventilation with production of the proper tensions of oxygen and carbon dioxide in alveolar gas can be of use to man only if the pulmonary capillary bed is perfused adequately and is exposed to this alveolar gas. The pulmonary blood flow and its distribution are therefore of vital importance.

The pulmonary circulation is a low-pressure system functioning with a mean pulmonary-artery pressure of 15 mm Hg and a mean left-atrial pressure of 5 mm Hg. This pressure differential of 10 mm Hg propels the pulmonary blood volume of approximately 900 ml in the healthy adult, through the circulation to the left atrium at a rate sufficient to allow the entire cardiac output to flow through the pulmonary circulation. Normally the resistance of the vascular bed in the lungs adapts readily to an increase in flow, as for example during exercise when pulmonary blood flow may double or triple without increase in mean pulmonary artery pressure.

In the healthy young adult removal of one-half of the pulmonary circulation by pneumonectomy does not result in a rise in pulmonary artery pressure even though the entire cardiac output is flowing through the remaining one-half of the pulmonary vascular bed. Increase in pulmonary artery pressure can result from increase in left atrial pressure secondary to valvular disease in the left heart, from increase in vasoconstriction which normally occurs with hypoxemia, from mechanical obstruction of pulmonary artery branches by emboli (vasospasm also probably is present), or from diseases of the vascular wall.

Ventilation-Perfusion Relationships

The match of ventilation and perfusion in all parts of the lung is extremely important. Ventilation of the lungs is usually somewhat uneven, the most active air flow being in the superior portions and the least active in the dependent portions. Pulmonary blood flow is influenced by gravity to the extent that in the upright position the superior one-third of the lung field receives very little flow, while the dependent one-third receives a disproportionately large flow. Some imbalance of ventilation and perfusion is thus normally present.

Imbalance of ventilation and perfusion is markedly accentuated in an injured patient as excursion of the lower thorax may be limited by pain or a surgical incision, and evacuation of mucous in the dependent tracheobronchial tree is inhibited by lack of the ability to cough. Unless these restrictive factors are treated or ventilation assisted, gross abnormalities of ventilation-perfusion may occur. This produces a waste of ventilation (increase in V_D) in areas where no blood is flowing, and a lack of oxygenation in areas where blood flows past nonventilated alveoli. Frequent changes in position are threfore important to improve ventilation and perfusion to all lung segments. Placement of incisions away from the upper abdomen and chest can improve postoperative respiratory function and restrictive bandaging must be avoided.

VENTILATION-PERFUSION IMBALANCE

In a normal lung with a normal ventilation-perfusion ratio of 0.8, blood emerging from the pulmonary veins will be maximally oxygenated except for the admixture of a small portion, approximately 7 per cent, which flows through nonventilated lung tissue. The P_aO_2, therefore, should be approximately 100 mm Hg while breathing room air at sea level. Decrease in overall ventilation will reduce alveolar oxygen and likewise reduce P_aO_2, even though the ventilation-perfusion ratio is normal. Alteration of the ventilation-perfusion balance allowing blood to flow past nonventilated alveoli such as occurs in pneumonitis and atelectasis will produce a decrease in P_aO_2 even in the presence of a normal alveolar minute volume. This decrease in P_aO_2 in the presence of normal oxygen tensions in the pulmonary alveoli is due to the admixture of properly oxygenated blood with poorly oxygenated blood and is termed pulmonary venoarterial shunting, or simply pulmonary shunting.

Pulmonary shunting increases the difference between pulmonary alveolar oxygen tension (P_AO_2) and systemic arterial oxygen tension (P_aO_2). Another cause of depressed P_aO_2 in the presence of normal P_AO_2 is diffusion block, caused by abnormality of the alveolar septa. In normal individauls the possibility that A–a O_2 difference may be due to difficulties in diffusion of gas from the alveolus to the blood may be removed by allowing the patient to breath 100 per cent oxygen for 15 minutes. One hundred per cent oxygen in the pulmonary alveoli will saturate the alveolar septa and allow arterial blood P_{O_2} to rise, even in the presence of some diffusion block. If the difference between P_AO_2 and P_aO_2 remains abnormally high after breathing 100 per cent oxygen, a significant pulmonary shunt is present. The amount of the shunt in per cent of cardiac output may be calculated by measuring the arterial and mixed venous P_{O_2} and applying the standard shunt equation (p. 18).

In individuals where changes in interstitial lung tissue may be present, including such problems as the septic or posttraumatic pulmonary insufficiency syndrome, even 100 per cent oxygen breathing may not overcome alveolar septal thickening. Some degree of diffusion block may remain. For this reason 30 minutes of 100 per cent oxygen breathing is used as a test for pulmonary shunting, and results must be carefully interpreted.

METHODS FOR EVALUATION OF RESPIRATORY FUNCTION

The development of membrane electrodes for the rapid measurement of gas tensions of oxygen and carbon dioxide in blood and other fluids has provided the clinician with a powerful tool for the evaluation of respiratory function. Together with the rapid-reading pH electrode, blood-gas analysis provides fast, accurate, and repeatable measurements to guide in evaluation of function and response to therapy. Blood-gas analysis should be available whenever major surgery is undertaken, major trauma is treated, or the seriously medically ill patient is given care.

Arterial Blood Gases

P_aO_2

The net effects of function of the respiratory apparatus and the appropriateness of ventilation and perfusion are seen in P_aO_2 levels. If P_aO_2 is normal while breathing room air, the respiratory apparatus is functioning adequately for basal needs. If P_aO_2 remains normal following exercise, ventilatory reserve is good. If P_aO_2 is abnormally low, below 70 mm Hg at sea level, further studies should be done.

P_aCO_2

P_aCO_2 values should be at normal levels. Elevation of the P_aCO_2 above 40 mm Hg is an indication of respiratory insufficiency and/or hypoventilation. In a study by Stein et al [1-5] all patients with preoperative elevation of P_aCO_2 developed pulmonary complications after operation. Exercise tolerance using one to two flights of stairs with monitoring of vital signs and postexercise blood gases can be used as a practical test for cardiopulmonary reserves.

Studies of Ventilation

TOTAL FORCED VITAL CAPACITY

The simplest studies are the total forced vital capacity (FVC), the maximal expiratory flow rate (MEFR), and the forced expiratory volume in one second (1^sVC). These studies can be done using an inexpensive spirometer. Approximate normal values for vital capacity can be determined by the following formula:

$$\text{For males:} \quad VC = [27.63 - (0.112 \times \text{age})]\ ht,\ cm$$
$$\text{For females:} \quad VC = [21.78 - (0.101 \times \text{age})]\ ht,\ cm$$

MAXIMAL EXPIRATORY FLOW RATE

Maximal expiratory flow rate is related to the ability to cough, and can be a good indication of the ability to clear the airway. The normal value is >200 liters/min (>300 liters/min in patients less than age 40) [1-6]. Stein and co-workers classified patients by this test preoperatively and showed an incidence of pulmonary complications of 3 per cent in normals (mean 280 liters/min) and of 70 per cent in those with reduced MEFR (mean 110 liters/min) [1-5].

FORCED EXPIRATORY VOLUME IN ONE SECOND

The normal value for the forced expiratory volume in one second is 70 per cent of the total vital capacity or more.

PULMONARY SHUNT MEASUREMENT

Estimation of pulmonary shunt can be made by measurement of P_aO_2 after 30 minutes of 100 per cent oxygen breathing. The amount of the functional pulmonary shunt may be calculated using a formula derived from the original one proposed by Rahn and Farhi [1-7]. The commonly used formula is

$$\frac{Q_s}{Q_t} = \frac{(P_A - P_a) \times 0.0031}{(C_a - C_v) + [(P_A - P_a) \times 0.0031]}$$

where Q_s = shunt flow

Q_t = cardiac output

P_A = alveolar oxygen tension

P_a = arterial oxygen tension

C_a = arterial oxygen content

C_v = mixed venous oxygen content

In general it has been shown that a P_aO_2 below 500 mm Hg after 30 minutes of 100 per cent oxygen breathing suggests an increase in pulmonary shunt above normal. A P_aO_2 of 300 to 400 mm Hg is associated with a 10 to 20 per cent shunt and a P_aO_2 of 100 mm Hg or less with a shunt of 30 to 50 per cent of cardiac output.

In complicated situations, especially if pulmonary resection is to be performed, complete pulmonary function tests by a pulmonary function laboratory should be done.

PREOPERATIVE EVALUATION

Careful appraisal of the adequacy of respiratory function must be made in any patient about to undergo an operation. Careful physical examination and chest x-ray may be sufficient in young patients without prior history of lung disease. However, in any patient with prior history of lung disease, and in most patients over 50 years of age, evaluation of respiratory function should be done. Most important in the history is the presence of dyspnea, cough with sputum, and inhalation of tobacco smoke. All such patients should have, in addition to chest x-ray, an exercise test and a postexercise arterial blood-gas determination. If blood-gas values are normal and exercise tolerance is good, the patient is a good risk. However, if P_aO_2 levels are decreased below 100 mm Hg and exercise tolerance is poor, other studies should be done. These include the vital capacity, maximal expiratory flow rate, and forced expiratory volume in one second. If the forced expiratory volume in one second is decreased below 70 per cent of the tidal volume, inhalation of isoproterenol aerosol, 0.5 per cent, should be given and the forced expiratory volume repeated. Improvement in this percentage indicates bronchospastic disease and the need for pre- and postoperative bronchodilator therapy.

Measurement of the per cent of pulmonary shunt may be important in patients with emphysema or pulmonary fibrosis. Such patients have an increased admixture of unsaturated blood with a larger than normal difference between alveolar and arterial P_{O_2} [1-8]. Markedly obese patients also show an increased shunt percentage—a feature, however, that can be improved by deep respirations.

Preoperative Preparation

Patients who show a decrease in normal respiratory function by these tests should have preoperative therapy to include discontinuation of smoking, antibiotics as indicated by sputum cultures, bronchodilator drugs, postural drainage, and chest physiotherapy with special attention to deep breathing and coughing [1-9]. The use of proper preoperative preparation has reduced postoperative pulmonary complications in such patients [1-10]. In addition, the complications that do occur in the prepared patient are less severe than those occurring in comparable patients who do not receive similar preoperative preparation.

INTRAOPERATIVE CARE

During operation all patients must have respiratory function monitored to insure adequate oxygenation and removal of carbon dioxide. The simplest and surest method is the measurement of blood gases. P_aO_2 measurement gives information as to oxygen delivery into the blood, but may not be needed or indicated except in specific situations of known pulmonary insufficiency. Also, anesthetized patients are usually breathing oxygen-enriched gas mixtures. P_vCO_2 and mixed venous pH, obtained through a central venous catheter, can usually give sufficient information as to adequacy of ventilation [1-11]. Such sampling can be done easily and frequently during a surgical procedure, and should be routine in cases of major surgery, in aged patients, and in patients with known pulmonary disease.

Regional Anesthesia

Routine measurement of blood gases in patients under spinal and under local anesthesia has shown frequent periods of hypoventilation with hypercapnia and respiratory acidosis, unsuspected by the appearance of the patient. In the elderly patient under regional anesthesia, blood-gas analysis should be done at intervals during operation and all such patients should be urged to take frequent deep breaths.

General Anesthesia

The danger of hypoxemia and hypercapnia with respiratory acidosis at the time of apnea during anesthetic induction and endotracheal intubation has been stressed [1-12]. Two minutes of apnea without prior hyperventilation result in a significant rise in P_aCO_2 and fall in pH. This change in patients with abnormal cardiac irritability may result in serious arrhythmias or bradycardia with arrest. It is important to hyperoxygenate prior to endotracheal intubation and to limit the period of apnea to 60 seconds or less.

Patients under general anesthesia usually have respirations assisted or controlled by the anesthesiologist. With controlled respirations, it has been shown that normal respiratory minute volumes allow a gradual decrease in lung compliance and a progressive fall in P_aO_2, even when arterial pH and P_aCO_2 remain within normal limits [1-13]. Passive hyperinflation of the lung readily returns compliance to normal and raises P_aO_2 to proper levels. Presumably these changes are due to the development of atelectasis even with normal respiratory minute volumes. These factors demonstrate the importance of passive inflation of the lung to full expansion at regular intervals during general anesthesia.

Hyperventilation Dangers

Continued hyperventilation can maintain P_aO_2 at normal levels. However, P_aCO_2 will fall and pH rise indicating respiratory alkalosis. Cerebral blood flow decreases under these conditions and brain damage may result [1-14]. It has also been shown that sustained hyperventilation causes a loss of carbon dioxide stores from the body. Following cessation of prolonged hyperventilation, if the patient breathes room air, P_aCO_2 may remain subnormal because CO_2 is returning to the depleted storage sites. Hypoventilation occurs, since P_aCO_2 does not rise normally to stimulate an increase in ventilation. Such hyperventilation *with room air* causes a fall in P_aO_2 that may reach hypoxic levels. This danger is present especially in the first hour following cessation of anesthesia and hyperventilation, during return to spontaneous respirations with room air. Under these conditions a normal P_aCO_2 may not indicate normal alveolar ventilation. Thus hyperventilation during anesthesia may be undesirable and careful monitoring of the patient following resumption of spontaneous respirations is needed. The routine administration of oxygen is an important adjunct at this time [1-15].

Inability of the anesthesiologist to maintain a normal blood-gas profile should immediately trigger a logical investigation. Mild hypercapnia may be the result of hypoventilation, and more adequate exchange may be all that is necessary. If abnormalities occur despite seemingly adequate ventilation, the patient should be disconnected from any anesthetic apparatus and breathed with room air, using mouth-to-tube or Ambu bag respirations. Placement of the tube should be checked by auscultation of both sides of the chest. If air movement through the tube is at all difficult, the balloon should be deflated; if this does not provide immediate relief the tube should be rapidly removed and a new tube inserted.

Partial plugging of the tube with blood or secretions may cause elevation of P_aCO_2 with normal P_aO_2 being maintained as long as oxygen is administered. Ventilation seems normal under these circumstances, and suction catheters may pass easily through the small remaining lumen. Persistent elevation of the P_aCO_2 without obvious reason, therefore, mandates removal of the tube for inspection and replacement.

POSTOPERATIVE CARE

Attention to the adequacy of respiration is especially vital in the immediate postoperative period. Following cessation of controlled ventilation, spontaneous respiration occurs when P_aCO_2 rises above normal levels of 40 mm Hg. Anesthetic and narcotic drugs can depress the medullary respiratory center and decrease the ventilatory response to hypercapnia. The rise in P_aCO_2 and fall in pH may then set the stage for serious or fatal cardiac arrythmias [1-16]. In addition, hypoventilation at normocapneic levels may occur if body carbon dioxide stores have been depleted by prolonged hyperventilation.

The Decision to Extubate

The patient must be observed carefully with the endotracheal tube in place and minute ventilation estimated by observing the rate and depth of respirations. A maximum-flow-rate meter may be used to assess the return of adequate ventilation and cough strength. Arterial blood-gas tensions will corroborate the efficiency of respiratory action. The endotracheal tube must be maintained in place until the patient is ventilating adequately and is sufficiently alert to clear his own secretions. Following suction aspiration of mucous from the trachea and removal of the endotracheal tube, the adequacy of ventilation *must be proved* by careful observation of rate and depth of breathing and sequential arterial blood-gas studies.

The decision as to when it is safe to remove the endotracheal tube is a most difficult one, and if any question persists the tube should remain in place. Active motion of the patient to remove his own tube is not a sufficient sign of adequate breathing ability; patients have been seen who developed postextubation hypoxia and cardiac arrest after removing the tube spontaneously. *The only proof of adequate ventilation is a normal blood-gas profile.*

CHANGES IN RESPIRATION DUE TO SURGERY AND TRAUMA

Following surgery or trauma to the chest and abdomen, pulmonary compliance decreases and work of breathing increases. This is demonstrated clinically by increase in the respiratory rate [1-17, 1-18]. Such patients show a rise in respiratory work, a rise in minute volume, and a rise in the work/ventilation ratio with a decrease in lung compliance. Respiratory work is greater preoperatively in obese patients and is significantly increased in those patients postoperatively. Postoperative respiratory work is increased more in the elderly patient and after prolonged anesthesia. Studies measuring the forced expiratory volume in one second have shown marked decrease following abdominal and thoracic surgery [1-19]. The reduction in the ability to rapidly expire air ranged up to 50 per cent in upper abdominal surgery and returned to normal after one week in uncomplicated cases. Lower-abdominal incisions produced less alteration in breathing ability. It is thus apparent that a measurable reduction in pulmonary function occurs in patients who have undergone thoracic and abdominal operations. These changes predispose to ventilatory inadequacy, pooling of secretions, atelectasis, and pulmonary infections.

PULMONARY COMPLICATIONS

Proper care of the postoperative or posttrauma patient requires careful observation of respiratory function and a knowledge of the problems which may arise. An understanding of the frequent occurrence of serious respiratory insufficiency in the elderly, in patients with chronic lung disease, in patients following severe trauma, and in patients suffering from certain types of illness such as sepsis, pancreatitis, and liver disease, will alert the surgeon if the early signs of such insufficiency are known [1-20]. The basic requirements for adequate respiratory function are the provision of an open tracheobronchial tree, properly cleared of secretions by the patient or by expert tracheobronchial suctioning, the adequacy of respiratory minute ventilation produced spontaneously or by assistance from a mechanical respirator, and the proper amount and distribution of perfusion, determined by an adequate cardiac output and by frequent change of position to perfuse all lung segments in turn.

Respiratory Distress Syndrome

In a number of cases these rather simple methods are not sufficient to maintain adequate respiratory function because of the development of a diffuse pulmonary syndrome characterized by a falling P_aO_2 in the presence of adequate airway oxygen and minute alveolar ventilation. This variety of pulmonary insufficiency is characterized by an increasing pulmonary shunt and may develop after a wide variety of illness or injury. Such patients usually have severe problems of multiple trauma, multiple transfusions, sepsis, shock, or metabolic disturbances such as acute pancreatitis and liver failure [1-21].

First noticed is hyperventilation with respiratory alkalosis [1-22, 1-23, 1-24]. At this time, most of these patients do not have sufficient hypoxemia to cause hyperventilation ($P_aO_2 > 70$ mm Hg), and the etiology of the hyperventilation is obscure. The suggestion has been made that it is due to poor perfusion of the receptor cells in the aortic and carotid bodies with stimulation of respiration, even in the presence of normal P_aO_2. Another suggested etiology is that changes in the pulmonary stretch reflex (Hering-Breuer) may result from alterations in the composition of the pulmonary interstitium. Along with hyperventilation there is a decrease in lung compliance and an increase in the work of breathing. Over the next 12 to 24 hours an increasing pulmonary shunt appears with fall in P_aO_2. Increase in airway oxygen is required to prevent significant hypoxemia. As the pulmonary shunt increases, cardiac output rises as a response to open vascular beds in hypoxic tissues. If cardiac function fails to sustain the hyperdynamic state in the face of an increasing pulmonary shunt, the circulation slows, metabolic acidosis appears, and the patient succumbs to cardiac arrhythmia and arrest.

Examination of the lungs of such patients at autopsy has shown patchy areas of consolidation with increased amounts of blood. These lungs contain more water and protein than normal [1-25]. Microscopically, edema of the interstitial tissues and capillary congestion are seen. Intra-alveolar pulmonary edema, atelectasis, and infection may also be present. Hyaline membranes are also seen [1-26].

The respiratory distress syndrome has a number of possible causes:

VENTILATION-PERFUSION IMBALANCE

Perfusion of unventilated alveoli seems to be the underlying cause of the large alveolar arterial P_{O_2} gradient. Atelectasis may be due to pooling of secretions, alteration in mucous production, interference with action of ciliated epithelial cells, or alterations in surfactant function.

ENDOTHELIAL DAMAGE AND INTERSTITIAL EDEMA

Damage to pulmonary endothelial cells may be the result of a variety of circulating substances and probably occurs in such states as prolonged shock, pancreatitis, severe sepsis, and liver damage. Teplitz [1-2], using chemical poisons, has shown progressive changes in endothelial cells of experimental animals with the production of a leak of fluid into the interstitial areas of the lung. Perivascular edema occurred and platelet thrombi blocked pulmonary capillaries. Such blockage by platelet thrombi and other debris has been demonstrated following shock [1-27] and trauma [1-28, 1-29].

OVERADMINISTRATION OF CRYSTALLOID FLUID

The administration of large amounts of crystalloid solution intravenously in the presence of this type of pulmonary capillary abnormality can result in leakage of fliud into the pulmonary interstitium [1-30]. If plasma proteins are diluted, further fluid transudation occurs due to the decrease in colloid osmotic pressure [1-31, 1-32]. Under these conditions, fluid leak may occur in the presence of a normal central venous pressure. Once such fluid transudation begins, the accumulation of fluid may occur at an increased rate for reasons not completely understood. At this stage the patient may show tachypnea without moisture being audible on auscultation of the chest. X-ray examination, however, shows diffuse opacification of the lung fields, and is the most important diagnostic finding.

OXYGEN TOXICITY

Oxygen itself has been implicated in the production of the pathologic changes present in this diffuse lung lesion. It is thought that pulmonary damage is related not only to the level of oxygen in the inspired air, but to the P_aO_2 with less damage occurring if the P_aO_2 is not markedly elevated [1-33]. Other studies have suggested that a normal P_aO_2 does not protect against such damage [1-34]. Six to 12 hours of inhalation of 100 per cent oxygen is apparently not damaging to normal man [1-35], and up to 21 hours of such exposure caused no measurable change in postcardiotomy patients [1-36]. Longer exposure (>30 hrs) to 100 per cent oxygen in patients has been shown to produce lowering of P_aO_2, increase in pulmonary shunting, increase in V_D/V_T ratio, and increase in lung weights [1-37]. The effect of such elevated oxygen tensions on the possibly altered interstitium found in some patients is still unknown. Oxygen tensions below 60 per cent ($P_AO_2 < 400$ mm Hg) appear to be safe. The importance of measurement of the actual oxygen tension used with mechanical respiration has been repeatedly stressed [1-38, 1-39], and erroneously high concentrations of oxygen may be administered if this is not done.

REFLEX EFFECTS

A specific type of pulmonary edema appears to occur following head injury [1-40], and in association with increased intracranial pressure [1-41]. This occurs suddenly and appears to be mediated through a massive sympathetic discharge shifting blood from the periphery to the pulmonary circuit.

Pulmonary Embolization

Respiratory insufficiency may also be produced by embolization of the pulmonary arteries by gross clot or due to diffuse involvement by fat emboli. The diagnosis of massive pulmonary embolization may not be difficult due to the suddenness of onset of symptoms and the usual elevation of right heart pressures as determined by the central venous catheter [1-42, 1-43]. However, the frequency of small, multiple pulmonary emboli, especially in the aged and in patients after operation and trauma, may be much higher than is clinically recognized [1-44]. Confirmation of diagnosis should be made by pulmonary angiography and/or lung scan.

Fat Embolization

Embolization of the pulmonary arterial tree by fat may also be a relatively frequent occurrence. The diagnosis can usually be made if the lesion is considered [1-45]. The symptoms usually are those of respiratory insufficiency and/or mental confusion, with petechiae commonly seen. The P_aO_2 is usually depressed. There may be elevation of the central venous pressure and diffuse haziness with evenly distributed small fleck-like shadows in the chest x-ray [1-46, 1-47]. It has been suggested that much of the mental clouding seen in these patients may be due to hypoxia, and that the mental state may improve with appropriate oxygen therapy. The association of fat embolization with fall in the hematocrit has been noted by several authors, and the suggestion has been made that improvement in resuscitation may reduce the incidence of fat embolization [1-47].

Pulmonary Burns

Direct chemical injury to the tracheobronchial tree can occur following thermal burn, especially where burns of the face and oral cavity are noted. However, the development of diffuse pulmonary clouding on the chest x-ray and the syndrome of progressive pulmonary insufficiency in these patients may indicate a generalized phenomenon in addition to the local injury. The marked loss of resistance to infection in the massively burned patient increases the danger of severe pneumonia. An average mortality of nearly 50 per cent in pulmonary thermal injury indicates the severity of the problems encountered [1-48].

Aspiration of Gastric Contents

Aspiration of gastric contents may be another significant feature in the extremely ill patient. Such aspiration may occur in any patient who is unconscious or whose reflexes are depressed by narcotics, shock, or anesthesia. Distention of the upper gastrointestinal tract is a predisposing factor. Silent aspiration may be undetected and yet occur in as many as 16 per cent of cases when the patient is unconscious [1-49]. Asphyxia may occur immediately if large amounts of fluid or solid matter are aspirated. The more common aspiration, however, may be that of small amounts of gastric content.

The effect on the pulmonary and bronchial tissues appears to be dose-related. Small amounts of gastric acid introduced into the tracheobronchial tree produce hyperventilation and hypocapnia but not hypoxemia. Larger amounts produce massive outpouring of frothy blood tinged fluid into the tracheobronchial lumen, with fall in the P_aO_2. Chest x-ray usually will show diffuse opacification developing over a period of several hours [1-50].

GUIDELINES FOR THERAPY

Evaluation

Survival of the patient suffering from the diffuse type of pulmonary insufficiency syndrome will depend on the early detection of changes and careful application of therapy [1-51]. The patient should be monitored by frequent blood-gas analysis, measurement of serum electrolytes and protein, daily weighing, measurements of the central venous pressure, and careful intake and output recording. Restrictions in amounts of crystalloid infusion should be made, and early and frequent chest x-rays should be taken to detect interstitial fluid, which is *undetectable by physical examination in the early stages.*

The onset of tachypnea with respiratory alkalosis is the indication for careful monitoring. Decrease in the vital capacity, or the appearance of significant A–a O_2 deficit indicate the need for specific therapy. The intent of therapy is to maintain P_aO_2 at a level of 70 mm Hg, and if possible to prevent the pulmonary shunt from rising above 40 per cent, as this is associated with an increased mortality [1-52]. If assistance or control of respirations is required, an indwelling endotracheal tube should be used if the assistance is for only one or two days, as avoidance of tracheostomy is preferable. However, if assistance is required for a longer period, tracheostomy should be done. The dangers of tracheal damage from occlusive balloons on endotracheal tubes and tracheostomy tubes should be kept in mind, and soft balloons or loose inflation used [1-53, 1-54]. Tracheal damage if it occurs may cause stenosis and require later correction [1-55].

Respiratory Assistance

Control of respirations should be maintained using a respiratory pattern of slow deep respirations which improves alveolar minute volume and may in itself decrease pulmonary shunt. Periodic full inspiration with maintenance of the full expanded state for five seconds may reopen some alveoli and improve ventilation-perfusion dynamics [1-56]. Inspired oxygen concentrations should be regulated to produce a P_aO_2 of from 70 to 90 mm Hg.

Steroids

Corticosteroid administration seems to be beneficial in patients with pulmonary injury due to thermal burns [1-48], and should be used as early as possible in patients suffering from aspiration of acid gastric juice [1-57]. Prevention of fluid transudation into interstitium, alveoli, and bronchioles due to chemical damage is of utmost importance. Steroids may also be important in the therapy of massive fat embolism [1-58, 1-59]. In all of these conditions oxygen therapy with positive pressure ventilation is indicated [1-60].

Diuresis and Protein Infusion

If fluid transudation into interstitial tissues and pulmonary alveoli has taken place, the use of potent diuretics, such as ethacrynic acid or furosemide, combined with colloid infusion to raise intravascular colloidal pressure may be life-saving [1-61].

Positive-Pressure Breathing

In certain instances, continuous positive-pressure breathing by the use of expiratory retard, may produce improved arterial oxygen levels and be preferable to the use of intermittent positive pressure [1-62, 1-63]. Decrease in the percentage of pulmonary shunt has been noted with the use of this therapy. It should be remembered that pressure-controlled ventilators have far less controllability and require an increased work of breathing than volume-controlled respirators, and the volume-controlled type is required for continuous positive-pressure breathing [1-64].

Decrease in venous return to the heart with fall in cardiac output may occur with continuous positive pressure breathing if expiratory pressures are raised above 6 to 8 cm H_2O. Expiratory pressures up to 15 cm H_2O have been used successfully, however. The effect on cardiac output appears to be less when compliance has decreased. Careful monitoring is required.

Decrease in cardiac output has been noted with inspiratory pressures exceeding 20 mm Hg [1-65]. The net effect of increase in airway pressure to produce adequate ventilation and its effect on cardiac output must be assessed in determining the optimum pressures and rates to be used [1-66]. In some cases volume expansion to raise central venous pressure and restore right heart filling may be advantageous.

The fact that respirator therapy with hydrated air may produce water retention in the patient should not be overlooked. The inspiration of air 100 per cent saturated with water vapor blocks the normal respiratory excretion of water. This fact must be taken into consideration when calculating the fluid balance. Daily weights can be of considerable assistance and should be measured [1-67].

REFERENCES

1-1. Weibel, E. R., and Gomez, D. M.: Architecture of the human lung. Science 137:577, 1962.

1-2. Teplitz, C.: The ultrastructural basis for pulmonary pathophysiology following trauma. J. Trauma 8:700, 1968.

1-3. West, J. B.: Causes of carbon dioxide retention in lung disease. New Engl. J. Med. 284:1232, 1971.

1-4.   Dexter, L. (ed.): Aging of the lung. Perspectives, on biochemistry, immunology, stress, and lung function in relation to age. JAMA 186:24, 1963.

1-5.   Stein, M., Koota, G. M., Simon, M., and Frank, H. A.: Pulmonary evaluation of surgical patients. JAMA 181:765, 1962.

1-6.   Kory, R. C., Callahan, R., Boren, H. G., and Syner, J. C.: The Veterans Administration-Army cooperative study of pulmonary function. Am. J. Med. 30:243, 1961.

1-7.   Rahn, H., and Farhi, L. E., in Field, J. (ed.) Handbook of physiology: Sec. 3, Respiration. Washington, D.C., American Physiological Society, 1964, Vol. 1, p. 735.

1-8.   Said, S. I., and Banerjee, C. M.: Venous admixture to the pulmonary circulation in human subjects breathing 100 per cent oxygen. J. Clin. Invest. 42:507, 1963.

1-9.   Bendixen, H. H.: Respiratory Care. St. Louis, Mosby, 1965, pp. 93–103.

1-10.   Stein, M., and Cassara, E. L.: Preoperative pulmonary evaluation and therapy for surgery patients, JAMA 211:787, 1970.

1-11.   Phillips, B., and Peretz, D. I.: A comparison of central venous and arterial gas values in the critically ill. Ann. Intern. Med. 70:745, 1969.

1-12.   Medrado, V., and Stephen, C. R.: Arterial blood gas studies during induction of anesthesia and endotracheal intubation. Surg. Gynec. Obst. 123:1275, 1966.

1-13.   Bendixen, H. H., Hedley-Whyte, J., and Laver, M. B.: Impaired oxygenation in surgical patients during general anesthesia with controlled ventilation. New Engl. J. Med. 269:991, 1963.

1-14.   Shapiro, W., Wasserman, A. J., Baker, J. P., and Patterson, J. L., Jr.: Cerebrovascular response to acute hypocapnic and eucapnic hypoxia in normal man. J. Clin. Invest. 49:2362, 1970.

1-15.   Salvatore, A. J., Sullivan, S. F., and Papper, E. M.: Postoperative hypoventilation and hypoxemia in man after hyperventilation. New Engl. J. Med. 280:467, 1969.

1-16.   Osborn, J. J., Raison, J. C. A., Beaumont, J. O., Hill, J. D., Kerth, W. J., Popper, R. W., and Gerbode, F.: Respiratory causes of "sudden unexplained arrhythmia" in postthoracotomy patients. Surgery 69:24, 1971.

1-17.   Okinaka, A. J.: The pattern of breathing after operation. Surg. Gynec. Obst. 125:785, 1967.

1-18.   Neely, W. A., Robinson, T., McMullan, M. H., Bobo, W. O., Meadows, D. L., and Hardy, J. D.: Postoperative respiratory insufficiency: Physiological studies with therapeutic implications. Ann. Surg. 171:679, 1970.

1-19.   Bevan, P. G.: Factors affecting respiratory capacity in patients undergoing abdominal surgery. Brit. J. Surg. 214:126, 1961.

1-20. Peters, R. M., and Hilberman, M.: Respiratory insufficiency: Diagnosis and control of therapy. Surgery 70:280, 1971.

1-21. Collins, J. A.: The causes of progressive pulmonary insufficiency in surgical patients. J. Surg. Res. 9:685, 1969.

1-22. Lyons, J. H., Jr., and Moore, F. D.: Posttraumatic alkalosis: Incidence and pathophysiology of alkalosis in surgery. Surgery 60:93, 1966.

1-23. Berman, I. R., Moseley, R. V., Doty, D. B., and Gutierrez, V. S.: Posttraumatic alkalosis in young men with combat injures. Surg. Gynec. Obst. 134:11, 1971.

1-24. MacLean, L. D., Mulligan, G. W., McLean, A. P. H., and Duff, J. H: Alkalosis in septic shock. Surgery 62:655, 1967.

1-25. Gump, F. E., Mashima, Y., Ferenczy, A., and Kinney, J. M.: Pre- and postmortem studies of lung fluids and electrolytes. J. Trauma 11:474, 1971.

1-26. Webb, W. R.: Pulmonary complications of nonthoracic trauma: Summary of the National Research Council Conference. J. Trauma 9:700, 1969.

1-27. Allardyce, B., Hamit, H. F., Matsumoto, T., and Moseley, R. V.: Pulmonary vascular changes in hypovolemic shock: Radiography of the pulmonary microcirculation and possible role of platelet embolism in increasing vascular resistance. J. Trauma 9:403, 1969.

1-28. Berman, I. R., Gutierrez, V. S., Burran, E. L., and Boatright, R. D.: Intravascular microaggregation in the young men with combat injuries. Surg. Forum 20:14, 1969.

1-29. McNamara, J. J., Molot, M. D., and Stremple, J. F.: Screen filtration pressure in combat casualties. Ann. Surg. 172:334, 1970.

1-30. Adriani, J., Zepernick, R., Harmon, W., and Hiern, B.: Iatrogenic pulmonary edema in surgical patients. Surgery 61:183, 1967.

1-31. Gaar, K. A., Taylor, A. E., Owens, L. J., and Guyton, A. C.: Effect of capillary pressure and plasma protein on development of pulmonary edema. Am. J. Physiol. 213:79, 1967.

1-32. Levine, O. R., Mellins, R. B., Senior, R. M., and Fishman, A. P.: The application of Starling's law of capillary exchange to the lungs. J. Clin. Invest. 46:934, 1967.

1-33. Winter, P. M., Gupta, R. K., Michalski, A. H., and Lanphier, E. H.: Modification of hyperbaric oxygen toxicity by experimental venous admixture. J. Appl. Physiol. 23:954, 1967.

1-34. Miller, W. W., Waldhausen, J. A., and Rashkind, W. J.: Comparison of oxygen poisoning of the lung in cyanotic and acyanotic dogs. New Engl. J. Med. 282:943, 1970.

1-35. Van de Water, J. M., Kagey, K. S., Miller, I. T., Parker, D. A., O'Connor, N. E., Sheh, J., MacArthur, J. D., Zollinger, R. M., Jr., and Moore, F. D.: Response of the lung to six to 12 hours of 100 per cent oxygen inhalation in normal man. New Engl. J. Med. 283:621, 1970.

1-36.   Singer, M. M., Wright, F., Stanley, L. K., Roe, B. B., and Hamilton, W. K.: Oxygen toxicity in man. A prospective study in patients after open-heart surgery. New Engl. J. Med. 283:1473, 1970.

1-37.   Barber, R. E., Lee, J., and Hamilton, W. K.: Oxygen toxicity in man. A prospective study in patients with irreversible brain damage. New Engl. J. Med. 283:1478, 1970.

1-38.   Pontoppidan, H., and Berry, P. R.: Regulation of the inspired oxygen concentration during artificial ventilation. JAMA 201:11, 1967.

1-39.   Harris, T. M., Gray, M., Petty, T. L., and Mueller, R.: Monitoring inspired oxygen pressures during mechanical ventilation. JAMA 206:2885, 1968.

1-40.   Simmons, R. L., Martin, A. M., Jr., Heisterkamp, C. A., III, and Ducker, T. B.: Respiratory insufficiency in combat casualties: II. Pulmonary edema following head injury. Ann. Surg. 170:39, 1969.

1-41.   Berman, I. R., and Ducker, T. B.: Pulmonary, somatic and splanchnic circulatory responses to increased intracranial pressure. Ann. Surg. 169:210, 1969.

1-42.   Marshall, R.: Physiological disorders in pulmonary embolism. Brit. J. Surg. 55:794, 1968.

1-43.   DelGuercio, L. R. M., Cohn, J. D., Feins, N. R., Coomaraswamy, R. P., and Mantle, L.: Pulmonary embolism shock. JAMA 196:751, 1966.

1-44.   Morrell, M. T., and Dunnill, M. S.: The post-mortem incidence of pulmonary embolism in a hospital population. Brit. J. Surg. 55:347, 1968.

1-45.   Peltier, L. F.: The diagnosis of fat embolism. Surg. Gynec. Obst. 122:371, 1965.

1-46.   Rokkanen, P., Lahdensuu, M., Kataja, J., and Julkunen, H. The syndrome of fat embolism: Analysis of thirty consecutive cases compared to trauma patients with similar injuries. J. Trauma 10:299, 1970.

1-47.   Fuchsig, P., Brucke, P., Blumel, G., and Gottlob, R.: A new clinical and experimental concept on fat embolism. New Engl. J. Med. 276:1192, 1967.

1-48.   Stone, H. H., and Martin, J. D., Jr.: Pulmonary injury associated with thermal burns. Surg. Gynec. Obst. 130:1242, 1969.

1-49.   Culver, G. A., Makel, H. P., and Beecher, H. K.: Frequency of aspiration of gastric contents by the lungs during anesthesia and surgery. Ann. Surg. 133:289, 1951.

1-50.   Awe, W. C., Fletcher, W. S., and Jacob, S. W.: The pathophysiology of aspiration pneumonitis. Surgery 60:232, 1966.

1-51.   Wilson, R. F., Larned, P. A., Corr, J. J., Sarver, E. J., and Barrett, D. M.: Physiologic shunting in the lung in critically ill or injured patients. J. Surg. Res. 10:571, 1970.

1-52. Wilson, R. F., Kafi, A., Asuncion, Z., and Walt, A. J.: Clinical respiratory failure after shock of trauma. Arch. Surg. 98:539, 1969.

1-53. Grillo, H. C.: The management of tracheal stenosis following assisted respiration. J. Thorac. Cardiovasc. Surg. 57:52, 1969.

1-54. Bryant, L. R., Trinkle, J. K., and Dubilier, L.: Reappraisal of tracheal injury from cuffed tracheostomy tubes. JAMA 215:625, 1971.

1-55. Geffin, B., Grillo, H. C., Cooper, J. D., and Pontoppidan, H.: Stenosis following tracheostomy for respiratory care. JAMA 216:1984, 1971.

1-56. Ward, R. J., Danziger, F., Bonica, J. J., Allen, G. D., and Bowes, J.: An evaluation of postoperative respiratory maneuvers. Surg. Gynec. Obst. 124:51, 1966.

1-57. Lawson, D. W., Defalco, A. J., Phelps, J. A., Bradley, B. E., and McClenathan, J. E.: Corticosteroids as treatment for aspiration of gastric contents: An experimental study. Surgery 59:845, 1966.

1-58. Ashbaugh, D. G., and Petty, T. L.: The use of corticosteroids in the treatment of respiratory failure associated with massive fat embolism. Surg. Gynec. Obst. 124:493, 1966.

1-59. Fischer, J. E., Turner, R. H., Herndon, J. H., and Riseborough, E. J.: Massive steroid therapy in severe fat embolism. Surg. Gynec. Obst. 133:667, 1971.

1-60. Cameron, J. L., Sebor, J., Anderson, R. P., and Zuidema, G. D.: Aspiration pneumonia. Results of treatment by positive-pressure ventilation in dogs. J. Surg. Res. 8:447, 1968.

1-61. Skillman, J. J., Bushnell, L. S., and Hedley-Whyte, J.: Peritonitis and respiratory failure after abdominal surgery. Ann. Surg. 170:122, 1969.

1-62. Ashbaugh, D. G., Petty, T. L., Bigelow, D. B., and Harris, T. M.: Continuous positive-pressure breathing (CPPB) in adult respiratory distress syndrome. J. Thor. Cardiov. Surg. 57:31, 1969.

1-63. Ashbaugh, D. G.: Effect of ventilatory methods and patterns on physiologic shunt. Surgery 68:99, 1970.

1-64. Puryear, G. H., Osborn, J. J., Beaumont, J. O., and Gerbode, F.: The influence of adjuvant ventilators in the respiratory effort of acutely ill patients. Continuous measurement by digital computer. Ann. Surg. 170:900 1969.

1-65. McDonald, K. E., Camp, F. A., and Schenk, W. G., Jr.: A comparison of three mechanical ventilators. Arch. Surg. 87:796, 1963.

1-66. Kumar, A., Falke, K. J., Geffin, B., Aldredge, C. F., Laver, M. B., Lowenstein, E., and Pontoppidan, H.: Continuous positive-pressure ventilation in acute respiratory failure. New Engl. J. Med. 283:1430, 1970.

1-67. Sladen, A., Laver, M. B., and Pontoppidan, H.: Pulmonary complications and water retention in prolonged mechanical ventilation. New Engl. J. Med. 279:448, 1968.

2

ALIMENTARY TRACT

PRIMARY FUNCTION

"Nutrition is the science of food and its relation to health, and as such is inseparable from any concept of medicine." [2-1]

The alimentary tract is the mechanism for intake and absorption of most substrates for bodily metabolism. These include the three forms of fuel used by man: carbohydrate, fat and protein; the required minerals; the necessary vitamins; and the fluid intake appropriate to maintain homeostasis. Such normal intake is necessary to maintain health and is required to produce healing of traumatic or surgical wounds.

BODY COMPOSITION

Protein

The normal healthy human body is made up of protein, fat, carbohydrate, water, and minerals [2-2]. The protein content of the body is determined by the needs for those functions provided by protein and there is no excess protein pool [2-3]. Each protein molecule has a specific function, either as an enzyme, a structural component such as collagen, a contractile element such as actin or myosin, a means to provide oncotic pressure in the fluid spaces such as albumin, or to do many other things. The total protein content of the individual is thus determined by the internal regulatory systems for enzymatic and circulatory dynamics, and in part by the requirements for skeletal muscle mass which depend upon the level of daily exercise and activity.

Carbohydrate

Carbohydrate is stored in the body primarily as liver and muscle glycogen. The glycogen, in amounts of 50–75 gm for liver and approximately 200 gm for muscle, can provide only 12 hr of caloric need in itself. It is rapidly available for acute needs, however, and thus is utilized in emergency situations.

Fat

The fat content of the body exists primarily for energy storage. In certain locations fat also serves a mechanical function, as in the retroorbital, buccal, and periarticular locations. These fat deposits are protected from use as energy sources in times of depletion. The remainder of the body fat is stored in the subcutaneous and retroperitoneal areas and is available as an energy substrate.

NORMAL ENERGY REQUIREMENTS

The energy needs of the normal individual are determined by body size and levels of activity, and may be increased by the abnormal conditions of injury and wounding. A 70-kg man requires approximately 1800 calories per day to satisfy basal needs. Studies of normally active individuals have shown that from 2100 to 3700 calories per day can maintain normal nutrition over prolonged periods [2-4, 2-5]. Similar caloric needs have been documented using total intravenous alimentation [2-6].

Fate of Ingested Fuel Substances

The healthy individual on an adequate dietary intake, maintains an optimal protein mass determined by the normal state of exercise and the internal regulatory mechanisms regulating enzyme action and protein content of body fluid. Certain hormones such as androgens, insulin, and growth hormone are important in this regulation. Likewise, carbohydrate of the normal individual is maintained at optimal levels of liver and muscle glycogen. Excess calories, whether ingested as protein, carbohydrate, or fat, are therefore converted to fat and stored within the body in this available-energy pool. As Cahill has stated. "Fat . . . serves as man's caloric buffer with his environment, protein as his machinery, and carbohydrate reserves are spared for emergency use only." [2-3]

MALNUTRITION

Maintenance of this optimal condition is desirable to allow recovery from surgical trauma and to promote healing of surgical wounds. Any deficiency in caloric intake relative to the needs of body metabolism will permit utilization of endogenous tissues as body fuels. Although fat stores may be mobilized and consumed without interfering with the normal body economy, the conversion of endogenous protein immediately begins to alter the optimal body condition. Loss of skeletal muscle mass produces loss of strength and eventually causes severe weakness. Such loss of strength works against recovery as the patient may become unable to turn and cough effectively and too weak to move about normally.

Utilization of Endogenous Protein

Utilization of endogenous protein leads to a decrease in circulating albumin levels, reducing the osmotic pressure of the plasma. This in turn allows accumulation of edema fluid in body tissues which interferes with wound healing [2-7]. Changes in intestinal function due to hypoproteinemia and edema may perpetuate a vicious circle of starvation with loss of appetitie and interference with intestinal absorption of fuels. Increase in fluid "leakage" into other tissues, especially the lung interstitium and the brain, may seriously interfere with normal function [2-8, 2-9].

Effects on Wound Healing

Many studies have shown the adverse effects of malnutrition on the healing of wounds. As early as 1919 Clarke showed a decrease in wound healing in animals given deficient diets, especially diets deficient in protein [2-10]. Thompson and co-workers showed delayed healing of abdominal incisions with delay in normal fibroblastic proliferation [2-11]. Malnutrition appears to play a part in increasing the percentage of wound dehiscence [2-12, 2-13]. It has been suggested that this defect in healing is the result of deficiency of a specific amino acid such as methionine [2-14]. More recent studies, however, suggest that the deficiency is more complex and may involve multiple factors [2-15]. Alterations in other aspects of metabolic function may contribute to alteration in wound healing, as occurs in poorly controlled diabetic states [2-16].

Effects on Resistance to Infection

Normal metabolism and nutrition appear to be necessary to enable the body to resist invasive infection. A study of surgical wounds showed that infection occurred in 10.4 per cent of diabetic patients as compared to a normal expected rate of 7.4 per cent [2-17]. An increased incidence of wound infection was also seen in severely malnourished patients, although these patients tended to be older, with longer operations, and with a higher incidence of contaminated operations—all factors that increase wound infection. Extreme obesity contributed to an increase in the wound infection rate to 18 per cent. This was ascribed to the large amount of adipose tissue present, and the increased susceptibility of such tissue to invasive bacterial infection.

STARVATION

Study of the fasting normal human has provided information as to the preferential utilization of energy substrates. Benedict, in the first study of energy metabolism during starvation, noted that 75 per cent of the calories utilized were derived from fat [2-18]. Studies since then have determined that in a 24-hr period, a normal man consuming 1800 calories per day burns about 75 gm of protein, primarily from muscle, and 160 gm of adipose tissue triglyceride [2-4]. This normal endogenous requirement is satisfied by the oral feeding formula suggested by Randall of 35 calories per kilogram per 24 hr, with 1 gm of nitrogen for each 150 nonprotein calories [2-19]. The total caloric, protein, and nitrogen ratios suggested by Dudrick for intravenous feeding also closely follow this requirement [2-6]. In addition to calories and essential amino acids in protein, daily requirements of minerals, vitamins, and water have been determined [2-6, 2-19]. Metabolism of 75 gm of protein from muscle and 160 gm of adipose tissue triglyceride produces urinary losses approximating 10 to 15 gm of nitrogen daily.

Glucose Requirements of Fasting Man

Glucose, in excess of glycogen stores in liver or muscle, must be produced to supply brain metabolism. This need approximates 150 gm of glucose per day. Other glycolytic tissues—namely erthyrocytes, leukocytes, bone marrow, renal medulla, peripheral nerves, and some muscles—metabolize glucose but convert it to lactate and pyruvate. These substances are remade into glucose in the liver and kidney. Approximately 20 per cent of glucose utilized daily is converted in this manner.

The production of the required basal amount of glucose occurs in the liver where normal liver cells via enzymatic processes convert glycerol, lactate, pyruvate, and glucogenic amino acids into glucose [2-20]. The amino acids required for glyconeogenesis must come from the metabolism of body protein stores, predominantly striated muscle.

Protein Conservation by Fasting Man

As energy substrates, the other tissues of the body use either fatty acids released directly into the circulation or fatty acids partially oxidized to acetoacetate or beta-hydroxybutyrate (ketone bodies) by the liver. Conservation of body protein is thus accomplished by the utilization of adipose tissue triglycerides as the source of energy for a large part of the metabolic requirements. This fact makes it possible to block endogenous protein utilization in starving man by the administration of small amounts (100 gm/24 hr) of exogenous glucose.

Protein-Sparing Effect of Administered Glucose

The protein-sparing effect, noted many years ago by Gamble, occurs because the administered glucose provides the obligatory glucose substrate needed for brain metabolism and blocks gluconeogenesis from muscle-protein amino acids. Infusion of glucose stimulates insulin release which in turn appears to inhibit amino acid release from muscle, amino acid extraction by the liver, and glyconeogenesis from such amino acids as are extracted. Elevation of glucagon levels may also be involved in this regulation [2-21].

Although this amount of carbohydrate administered exogenously cannot prevent all of the glyconeogenesis from muscle protein, negative nitrogen balance falls from 10 to 15 gm to approximately 3 gm daily. The importance of providing at least 100 to 150 gm of glucose daily to the fasting individual is thus clear, as by this mechanism protein utilization as fuel is minimized. Semistarvation still continues, but with utilization of adipose tissue triglyceride from fat stores. Under normal conditions such fat stores can provide calories for a prolonged period of time.

Adaptation to Starvation

Total starvation for a period of more than a few days is associated with a change in brain metabolism in man. Although free fatty acids will not cross the blood-brain barrier due to binding to albumin, fatty-acid derived keto-acids cross this barrier readily, and are utilized to an increasing degree for brain fuel. The effect of adaptation of the brain to fat derived keto-acids is to decrease the requirement for glucose and thus decrease gluconeogenesis from muscle-protein amino acids. Under these conditions urinary nitrogen losses decreases to approximately 3 to 4 gm daily, an apparent irreducible minimum under the conditions of endogenous fuel utilization.

The exact mechanism by which brain metabolism alters it fuel source is not known, but appears to be regulated by insulin levels and perhaps by levels of alanine [2-3]. Prolonged starvation, therefore, reduces protein utilization to approximately 20 to 25 gm per day, representing 90 to 100 gm of wet muscle. In addition, the decrease in glyconeogenesis from amino acid leads to the production of less urea. Since urea is the primary solute in urine, obligatory urine water loss decreases during prolonged starvation, requiring less fluid intake.

INCREASE IN ENERGY REQUIREMENTS DUE TO SURGERY AND TRAUMA

Increase in energy requirements over basal levels may result from a variety of conditions encountered in surgical patients [2-22]. For many years, loss of body weight following surgical or accidental trauma has been noted.

Nitrogen Loss

Cuthbertson in 1932 was the first to measure excessive losses of nitrogen, sulfur, and phosphorus in patients who had sustained long-bone fractures [2-23]. Since those initial studies many authors have confirmed the excessive mobilization of body nitrogen following surgical trauma [2-24]. This occurs, for the most part, during the first three to fives days following injury, and varies according to the magnitude of the injury suffered. Studies have shown that the protein origin of this lost nitrogen is from the skeletal-muscle mass [2-25]. Total weight loss of 250 to 500 gm per day has been considered to be due to the effect of trauma itself [2-26]. By supplying adequate calories and nitrogen from exogenous sources, however, it has been possible recently to block the negative nitrogen balance usually seen following trauma [2-19, 2-27, 2-28, 2-29].

Effects on Stored Fat

Mobilization of fat stores with increase in free fatty acids has been shown to occur following injury [2-30]. When liver function is normal this elevation of plasma free fatty acid is transient, and returns to normal within 24 to 48 hr [2-31]. Release of free fatty acid into the circulation may cause hypercoagulability of blood due to platelet aggregation [2-32] or due to activation of certain clotting factors [2-33].

Causes of Tissue Catabolism

The exact cause of this increased catabolism has not yet been clearly identified. Studies by Kinney et al have shown that uncomplicated elective surgical operations are associated with a change of no more than ±10 per cent of the preoperative resting metabolic expenditure [2-34]. Their studies showed that metabolism of endogenous fat was directly related to the caloric deficit resulting from limited intake. Variations in protein and water loss occurred, however, with greater losses of both lean tissue and water in the male patient. It would thus appear that trauma results in selective mobilization of nitrogen for conversion to glucose.

Energy Requirements of the Wound

The energy requirements of the healing wound have been studied, and an increase in glucose uptake by the wound has been shown during the first three to four days after injury [2-35]. Glucose is also utilized by polymorphonuclear leukocytes, especially when exhibiting phagocytosis. Immature fibroblasts apparently receive their energy by glycolysis.

Energy Needs Due to Elevation of Body Temperature

The increase in energy requirement as a result of increase in body temperature has been studied by Kinney [2-36]. He and his group measured heat production of patients with varied types of trauma and found that increases in basal heat production after operation seldom exceeded 20 per cent of normal, and were found to exceed 50 per cent of normal only rarely, even after major trauma. The postoperative patient shows some degree of vasoconstriction, and heat loss may be diminished. Postoperative fever of low grade, not associated with infection, may be due to this slight rise in heat production with decrease in heat loss.

The early studies of DuBois showed a 7.2 per cent increase in caloric expenditure for every degree Fahrenheit increase in body temperature. This increase was the average figure for medical patients with infections or given pyrogenic injections [2-37]. In a series of 30 patients studied by Kinney, variations from the DuBois prediction were noted in most individuals. Some patients tended to show a less-than-expected rise in caloric expenditure with fever. These were usually the lethargic, obese, or elderly patient, especially females. Other patients showed a greater-than-predicted response to fever. These were the muscular, athletic, younger patients, particularly male. Patients suffering from major trauma showed an increase in energy expenditure greater than the DuBois formula in the first one to two weeks. Following this period, energy expenditure was reduced. Large third-degree burns or severe sepsis were associated with a sustained and high level of metabolic expenditure, at times reaching 160 to 180 per cent of the basal level [2-38].

Metabolic Requirements Due to Loss of Skin

A major proportion of the metabolic requirement of a patient with severe burns is the result of the evaporative water loss from burned skin. Roe et al have shown that large amounts of water may pass through the dry appearing third-degree burn eschar [2-39]. Studies by Jelenko et al showed that evaporative water loss through burn eschar averaged 298 gm/M²/hr when silver nitrate treatment was used, and 228 gm/M²/hr when sulfamylon was applied. Normal intact skin showed a water loss of 45 gm/M²/hr [2-40]. Each liter of water lost by evaporation requires an expenditure of approximately 580 calories in order to maintain a stable body temperature. Covering the burn eschar with an impermeable dressing can prevent this evaporative water loss and caloric expenditure. However, the prevention of all evaporative water loss may produce hyperthermia. The importance of early escharectomy and skin grafting in the reduction of the abnormally elevated metabolic requirement is therefore obvious [2-41, 2-42, 2-43].

Posttraumatic Carbohydrate Metabolism

Posttraumatic alteration in the metabolism of carbohydrate has been noted for some years [2-44]. Decreased carbohydrate tolerance has been shown in the immediate postoperative period [2-45]. This period, characterized as the adrenergic corticoid phase by Moore [2-24], is associated with an increase in the levels of many substances, including epinephrine, glucagon, growth hormone, thyroxin, and glucocorticoids. All of these hormones tend to increase blood-sugar levels and possibly inhibit carbohydrate utilization [2-46]. In addition, interference with insulin release has been suggested [2-47].

INTESTINAL FUNCTION

The intestinal tract prepares and absorbs fuel substances ingested with the aid of secreted acid, enzymes, and bile. Anatomically, the intestinal tract is suited for its function, with a large mucosal absorptive layer, the surface of which is extended through infolding and the presence of villi.

Stomach

Secretion of acid and pepsin occurs in the stomach with peptic digestion of protein occurring at pH of less than 3.5. The gastric wall also is the site of production of intrinsic factor which allows the absorption of vitamin B-12. The absence of large amounts of stomach reduces gastric secretion and inhibits B-12 absorption with the production of megaloblastic anemia. Postgastrectomy malabsorption of iron has also been noted.

Intestine

The duodenum and upper jejunum have been shown to be the most active parts of the intestine for the absorption of fat, carbohydrate, and protein [2-48]. Bypass of the duodenum by surgical creation of a gastro-jejunostomy is associated with decreased fat absorption [2-49]. Entry of sodium and water into the intestinal lumen occurs throughout the small intestine but is greatest in the duodenum.

CARBOHYDRATE ABSORPTION

Carbohydrate absorption can occur without the presence of sodium when concentrations within the lumen are higher than those in the serum. Active transport of glucose into the serum, however, has been shown to be sodium-dependent [2-50]. The sodium ion also is intimately involved with active water absorption [2-51, 2-52].

PROTEIN ABSORPTION

The protein within the intestine comes from ingested food and endogenous protein secretions. Between 10 and 30 gm of protein enter the lumen in secretions daily, and 250 gm of desquamated cells add another 25 gm of protein. Albumin from plasma proteins normally leaks into the intestine also [2-53]. Sixty per cent of fed protein is absorbed by the end of the duodenum, and all of the exogenous and endogenous protein is absorbed by the time it is transported to the terminal ileum. Protein is broken down into amino acids by the action of gastric pepsin and pancreatic trypsin prior to absorption.

FAT ABSORPTION

Absorption of fat is also carried out in the duodenum and jejunum. This requires a sequential procedure involving emulsification, hydrolysis, solubilization, adsorption, triglyceride resynthesis, chylomicron formation, and chylomicron transport [2-54]. Pancreatic lipase is essential for hydrolysis, and bile salts are essential for emulsification and transport. Fat is absorbed primarily in the form of fatty acids and monoglycerides, which are resynthesized to triglycerides within the mucosal cells. These fat droplets are then provided with a layer of phospholipid to form chylomicrons which enter the lymphatics for transport.

BILE ACIDS

Resorption of bile acids occurs by active transport in the ileum. Absence of the ileum almost completely interferes with this resorption [2-55] with resultant malabsorption of fat [2-56]. Malabsorption may occur due to deficient entry of bile into the intestine or from hepatic disease, and has been found in 50 per cent of patients with cirrhosis [2-57]. Steatorrhea is associated with deficiency of pancreatic lipase.

SHORT-BOWEL SYNDROME

Malabsorption may also occur due to marked shortening of the bowel. Studies on the surgical treatment of obesity have revealed that the function of 36 cm of jejunum and 10 cm of terminal ileum will allow constant slow weight loss on a limited diet. Dangers are deficiency of vitamins A and C and magnesium, and the development of fatty liver [2-58]. An occasional case with less remaining intestine has survived [2-59, 2-60, 2-61]. The syndrome itself is characterized by undernutrition, steatorrhea, and acidic diarrhea. This emphasizes the major problems, which are with absorption of fats and fat soluble materials due to interference with bile salt resorption [2-48], colonic diarrhea due to the presence of fatty acids and bile salts in the colon [2-62], and gastric hypersecretion [2-63]. Adaptation of the intestine occurs with time due to hypertrophy of intestinal villi [2-64] and increase in lining epithelial cells [2-65]. Treatment of the syndrome involves intravenous alimentation with gradual institution of easily absorbed oral feedings [2-66].

Colon

The function of the colon in man is to absorb sodium, chloride, and water brought into the colon from the terminal ileum, and to store the drier residue until it can be eliminated. Normally the colon absorbs 400 to 500 ml of water and 60 to 70 mEq of sodium per day, and secretes approximately 8 mEq of potassium a day [2-67]. Most of the resorption appears to occur in the right side of the colon. Colonic absorption is increased by the administration of mineralocorticoids and decreased by antidiuretic hormone. With salt deprivation the colon can increase sodium and water resorption. In the presence of inflammatory colonic diseases absorption is decreased. Abnormal secretion may occur in patients with villous adenoma. The colon appears to play a permissive role in the presence of small-bowel diarrhea, allowing diarrheal stools to be passed when the absorptive capacity of the colon is exceeded.

INTESTINAL BACTERIAL FLORA

Under normal conditions the human intestinal tract contains a relatively stable population of bacteria and fungi [2-68]. Viruses have not been isolated from intestinal contents, either from stomach [2-69] or intestine [2-70]. The jejunum is bacteriologically sterile in one-third of the subjects studied. Increasingly significant bacterial growth is obtained when the more distal ileum and colon are reached. Significant or resident bacteria are found in 100 per cent of colon specimens. This increase in resident microorganisms is true also of the fungal flora [2-71]. *Candida albicans* is obtained in 30 per cent of specimens of the oropharynx, in 54 per cent of specimens from the jejunum, in 55 per cent from the ileum, and in 65 per cent of fecal specimens. The relative stability of the bacterial flora of each normal individual has been shown by repetitive sampling over a period of several months.

Factors Controlling Growth of Intestinal Bacteria

The factors underlying the ability of the upper intestinal tract to limit bacterial growth are not clear. Within a few hours after the death of the host, bacterial infestation rapidly involves the entire length of the small intestine [2-72]. Alteration of this protective mechanism is present in cases of peritoneal sepsis, where extensive infestation of the upper small bowel by coliform bacilli is found [2-73]. Saliva apparently inhibits the growth of certain gram-positive bacteria [2-74], but other organisms such as *Streptococcus faecalis* and *Bacillus subtilis* live well in saliva [2-75]. Acid production by the stomach has been thought to maintain the sterility of the stomach and upper small intestine. The exact mechanism for this effect is still uncertain. Increased bacterial proliferation has been reported in patients with gastric retention, achlorhydria, cirrhosis, and following gastric resection [2-76].

The action of normal peristalsis may be the most important factor in moving bacteria to the distal portion of the intestine [2-77]. An overgrowth of bacteria occurs in situations which allow hypomotility of the bowel. Such failure of motility has been implicated in the bacterial overgrowth seen in sprue, intestinal diverticulosis, blind-loop syndrome, and in the afferent-loop syndrome following gastrectomy.

Normal Bacterial Content

The type of bacteria isolated from different parts of the intestinal tract varies considerably. *Escherichia coli* is found in 97 per cent of colonic specimens and is the most common aerobic organism. In the small bowel, gram-positive bacteria are more commonly seen. Anaerobic bacteroides are found in 83 per cent of stool specimens and are practically never seen in small-bowel aspirate. Alteration of the intraluminal bacterial population may be produced by changing the balance of bacterial growth with antibiotics. This may result in the production of staphlococcal or fungal enteritis. Decrease in the number of urea splitting organisms has been produced by an inoculum of *Lactobacillus* [2-78], a change which may reduce ammonia production in the colon. This therapy has been tried as a method of preventing encephalopathy in cirrhotic patients.

Bacterial Overgrowth

The presence of blind loops following small-bowel resection has allowed for bacterial overgrowth in some patients. Such bacterial proliferation can produce alteration in absorption of bile salts with abnormal absorption and steatorrhea resulting [2-79]. In addition, overgrowth of bacteria in blind loops has produced megaloblastic anemia due to deficiency in vitamin B-12 absorption [2-80, 2-81, 2-82].

ALTERATION IN INTESTINAL FUNCTION DUE TO TRAUMA

Alteration in the motor function of the intestine occurs following direct injury, physical handling, and exposure to the atmosphere during operation. Chemical irritation from acid gastric contents occurs following perforation of a peptic ulcer. The presence of localized or generalized infection adjacent to the bowel wall interferes with motility, and reflex inhibition of peristalsis results from retroperitoneal sepsis or injury. Failure of intestinal absorption and transport due to a variety of lesions is common experience in surgical practice. The "sentinel loop" of dilated small intestine present in some patients with pancreatitis is an example of such localized paralysis and malabsorption.

Ileus

Generalized ileus is seen after peritonitis, surgical intervention, direct trauma, or from distant effects such as renal calculi or fracture of the lumbar spine. The decrease in motility seen in a variety of types of ileus is apparently due to increase in inhibitory influences on the intestine rather than to lack of stimulatory mechanisms [2-83]. Blockade of the sympathetic outflow to the intestine has been used as a treatment for such ileus. Wright in 1935 used high spinal anesthesia to block sympathetic outflow activity [2-84]. The use of drugs to cause pharmacologic blockade of sympathetic activity is logical, and guanethidine has been effective in man [2-85].

Gastric Atony

It has been suggested that gastric atony may be more easily induced and may last for a longer period of time than intestinal atony [2-86, 2-87]. Such gastric stasis has been shown with and without vagotomy. Absence of sounds of small-bowel function in the postoperative period—the "silent postoperative abdomen"—may be due to lack of content, resulting from decrease in secretions and lack of entering volume. Rothnie et al showed that the normal sounds of the small bowel returned when fluid was placed in the jejunum [2-88]. Intestinal absorption can occur at a time when gastric atony precludes the emptying of material into the distal intestine. Wells et al used jejunal tube feedings successfully in 40 patients within 24 hours following gastrectomy [2-89]. Gastric distention must, therefore, be prevented by nasogastric suction following surgery and trauma. Material placed into the small intestine may be absorbed normally [2-90].

Effect of Intestinal Distention

In normal individuals the intestine contains small amounts of gas, 30 to 200 ml [2-91]. Usually nigrogen is the predominant gas. Oxygen is present in low concentrations (<2 per cent). Production of gas by intestinal bacteria (CO_2, H_2, and CH_4) is important in some individuals, and influences the entrapment of swallowed nitrogen in all individuals by reducing the luminal nitrogen partial pressure due to dilution. Distention of the small intestine appears to change absorption little until pressures over 60 to 70 cm H_2O are reached, when a decrease in absorption occurs. Secretion of fluid into the lumen increases as luminal pressure rises, accounting for the distention seen in "closed loop" obstructions [2-92]. In the colon, distention causes an increase in absorption with elevations up to 50 to 70 cm H_2O, following which absorption is decreased [2-93].

METHODS FOR EVALUATION OF INTESTINAL FUNCTION

Although function of the intestinal tract and associated organs is extremely complex, the evaluation of adequacy of intestinal function is based on a few simple observations. This may reflect the inability to measure many of the complex mechanisms which provide adequate nutrition. Clearly the most important assessment of adequacy of the entire system is a measurement of the patient's weight and an assessment of the general appearance. If the patient has been ingesting an adequate diet, the weight should be maintained and the muscle mass should be commensurate with the normal daily activity. Interference with normal nutrition may result from inability to ingest adequate fuel materials; from mechanical problems within the gastrointestinal tract; from lack of contact of foodstuffs with functioning intestine, the result of previous resection of bowel or intestinal bypass; and also from abnormalities of mucosal cell transport, abnormalities of intestinal lymphatic transport, and malfunction of associated organs such as pancreas and liver with failure of secretions to reach the intestinal lumen. In addition to these syndromes which are concerned primarily with absorption from the intestinal lumen into the bloodstream, common abnormalities of metabolism of the absorbed material may be present. These include specific enzyme deficiencies, diabetes, severe chronic liver disease, hyperthyroidism, and others.

General Assessment

The simplest and most direct assessment of nutritional state is a careful physical examination with attention to normality of appearance of skin and mucous membranes, evaluation of subcutaneous fat deposits, and assessment of muscle mass. Muscular strength and the ability of the patient to move about are directly related to the normal function of adequate muscle mass.

Basic Tests

Measurements of hemoglobin or hematocrit and of serum protein are indicated. The circulating protein may remain at relatively normal levels during progressive malnutrition as hemoglobin and circulating protein are selectively maintained until body stores are extremely depleted. Likewise, with replenishment of nutritional stores, hemoglobin and serum protein are first to be restored toward normal. A decreased level, therefore, without other cause, indicates severe protein depletion.

Measurements of liver function should be done and include measurement of the circulating enzymes, serum glutamic oxaloacetic transaminase (SGOT), serum glutamic pyruvic transaminase (SGPT), and lactic dehydrogenase (LDH), and the measurement of serum bilirubin and alkaline phosphatase. The presence of diabetes should be sought by measuring the fasting blood sugar or by the performance of a glucose tolerance test. Thyroid function is best assessed by physical examination followed by more specific tests if hyper- or hypothyroidism are suggested.

Tests of Absorption

If malnutrition is present and is not clearly explained by poor dietary intake, mechanical problems with the intestinal tract, obvious liver or pancreatic disease, or excessive intestinal losses due to inflammatory processes of the intestine, measurements of absorption are indicated.

FAT

Abnormal fat absorption with increased fecal fat losses may be diagnosed by inspection of the stool. If the stools are frequent, bulky, and pale, tending to float in water, increased fat loss is most certainly present. Proof of fat malabsorption can be obtained by measuring fecal fat. This is most reliably done by chemical analysis of a 72-hr stool collection according to the Van de Kamer method, with the patient ingesting 80 to 100 gm of fat per day. Under these circumstances, normal fat excretion is 5 gm or less per 24 hr [2-94]. This is a cumbersome method, however. An easily performed screening test for fat malabsorption is the serum carotene level. In the normal healthy individual the serum level is over 100 mcg/100 ml. Patients with malnutrition from reasons other than fat malabsorption usually have more than 50 mcg/100 ml of carotene in their serum. Those individuals with interference with fat absorption, however, will usually have values less than 20 mcg/100 ml [2-95].

CARBOHYDRATE

Sugar absorption can be measured by the xylose tolerance test. Xylose is a five-carbon sugar found in many fruits and vegetables. Normally at least one-half of a xylose load taken by mouth is absorbed and one-half of the amount absorbed is excreted in the urine. Xylose absorption takes place chiefly in the jejunum. The xylose tolerance test is performed by giving 25 gm of xylose by mouth. Urinary output of xylose usually exceeds 5 gm in the following five hours. Low excretion indicates disease of the upper small intestine or the presence of an inadequate absorbing surface, such as is found in the short-bowel syndrome. Xylose excretion is usually normal in pancreatic insufficiency [2-96].

Study of Anemia

The presence of an anemia which is out of proportion to the general nutritional deficiency indicates the need for special studies directed toward its cause. A search should be made for bleeding of gross or occult nature. Stool guaiac studies should be done on several occasions. A reticulocyte count should be performed.

IRON DEFICIENCY

Studies for iron deficiency should be carried out. Iron deficiency anemia may occur in the malabsorption states of adult celiac disease or granulomatous enteritis. Following subtotal gastrectomy approximately 50 per cent of patients show abnormal iron absorption from the gastrointestinal tract and may present with iron-deficiency anemia. In these patients the serum iron will be low, iron binding capacity will be high, and bone marrow will show little or no stainable iron.

B-12 ABSORPTION

Measurement of vitamin B-12 absorption should be done if iron deficiency anemia is ruled out. This is measured by the Schilling test. A small dose of radioactive vitamin B-12 is given by mouth, followed by 1 mg of nonradioactive B-12 injected parenterally. Under the influence of this B-12 load, radioactive vitamin B-12 is excreted in the urine. Normally the 24-hr excretion is 15 to 25 per cent of the ingested radioactive vitamin. Excretion of less than 5 to 8 per cent indicates malabsorption.

The separation of patients who lack production of intrinsic factor (i.e., those with pernicious anemia) from those who have intestinal malabsorption may be accomplished by a second test with radioactive vitamin B-12, this time administering intrinsic factor with the ingested dose. This combination will produce normal absorption in patients with pernicious anemia. This second test may remain abnormal in the presence of bacterial overgrowth such as found in blind-loop syndrome, patients with abnormalities of the ileal mucosa, or absence of distal ileum. In those patients with blind-loop syndrome and bacterial overgrowth, the administration of intestinal antibiotics will reverse an abnormal Schilling test to normal.

RED CELL MASS

A specific abnormality of the red blood cell mass of great importance to the surgeon may occur in patients who have suffered malnutrition for significant periods of time or who have been jaundiced for over two weeks. In these patients the hematocrit and hemoglobin levels may be only slightly diminished. However, the total blood volume may be contracted and the red blood cell mass abnormally low. Such patients should have blood-volume determinations performed using radioisotope techniques. Detection of an abnormally low blood volume is an indication for transfusion of whole blood or washed red cells.

Jejunal Mucosal Biopsy

Biopsy of the jejunal mucosa using the suction biopsy tube will allow a specific diagnosis of certain types of intestinal disease. Characteristic findings have been described in adult celiac disease, tropical sprue, Whipple's disease, lymphoma, amyloidosis, and diffuse nongranulomatous ileojejunitis [2-96].

PREOPERATIVE PREPARATION

Optimal recovery from surgical procedures requires restoration of nutrition to as normal a state as possible preoperatively. Moore has stated, ". . . Good feeding of good foods to good functioning gastrointestinal tracts is the key to recovery." [2-26] Diabetes must be well controlled, thyroid function returned to normal, and tissue catabolism prevented. If possible, actual reversal of a catabolic state with deposition of lean body tissue should be sought. In the functional malabsorptive states, this requires specific treatment for the absorptive abnormality.

Supplemented Oral Intake

In patients such as those with mechanical intestinal problems, short-bowel syndrome, or intestinal bypass; in those with abnormal losses due to chronic inflammatory disease of the intestine; and in patients with elevated caloric requirements (infections, burns, and the like), oral therapy should be tried. Oral feeding may be supplemented using low bulk dietary materials such as the recently available elemental diet [2-19]. This material may be administered by mouth, through a feeding tube, or by gastrostomy. As much as 5000 calories per day may be ingested in this manner with good intestinal tolerance and the need for small colonic evacuations only every five to six days. This would seem to be an ideal therapy for those patients with an intact and functioning intestinal tract.

Intravenous Alimentation

Intravenous alimentation should be used in those patients where the intestinal tract is not available for absorption or where intestinal function is altered by peritoneal infection; in patients where alimentary feeding is contraindicated due to intestinal fistulae; or in patients who require increased calories above those possible to ingest through the intestinal tract.

Nutritional support via a parenteral route has been attempted for many years. Whipple and his associates showed that intravenous plasma as the sole protein source could maintain normal nutrition in an animal receiving no protein by mouth [2-97]. This fact was confirmed by Allen et al in 1956 [2-98]. Rice and co-workers were able to provide total nutrition by vein for short periods (three to five days) using glucose, amino acids, and alcohol [2-99]. These authors felt that the nutritional support of surgical patients should consist of glucose, amino acids, calories, vitamins, electrolytes, and fluids, and that a positive nitrogen balance was desirable. With their regime they noted that patients so treated felt better, wounds healed more rapidly, less discomfort was suffered, ambulation was easier, and there was a shorter postoperative convalescence at home. The intravenous infusion of fat emulsions has been attempted for many years [2-100], and by some authors has been considered a practical means of administering calories parenterally [2-101].

The earlier attempts to supply nutrition by vein were largely ignored by most surgeons. It was not until Dudrick and co-workers reported longterm total nutrition in animals [2-102] and in humans [2-103, 2-104], that total parenteral nutrition became an accepted method of therapy. The development of this method has made it possible to reverse the catabolic state and initiate anabolism in extremely ill patients. This technique has been found valuable in patients with intestinal fistulae [2-105], in patients with renal failure [2-106], and in seriously ill infants and adults with a variety of problems [2-107, 2-108]. The possibility of long-term nutritional maintenance by this means may now be realized [2-109, 2-110].

INTRAOPERATIVE CARE

If the patient has been prepared properly, he should approach the operative experience with a normal body composition and the appropriate energy resources needed for a successful outcome. The intraoperative maintenance of nutritional support may not be warranted because of other considerations of fluid replacement. Loss of red blood cell mass due to bleeding must clearly be replaced. Resumption of intravenous alimentation where indicated should occur after the acute changes of the operative experience have resolved, usually within a matter of hours.

POSTOPERATIVE CARE

In the postoperative period, routine surgical care at present gives little attention to maintenance of normal nutrition. Most patients with operations of more routine magnitude regain intestinal function within two to three days, and the intake of body fuels reaches normal levels shortly thereafter. The routine administration of intravenous fluids, usually 5 per cent dextrose in water, provides 100 to 150 gm of glucose daily (2000 to 3000 ml of solution). This amount of glucose is capable of exerting the "protein-sparing effect" previously noted, and will limit the negative nitrogen balance to approximately 3 to 4 gm per day.

Patients with preexisting nutritional defects, patients whose surgical condition will preclude alimentation for more than three to four days, and patients who are experiencing large demands for energy production including those with major sepsis and burns should be placed on full nutritional maintenance using oral administration when possible, and otherwise employing intravenous alimentation. Special attention should be paid to the maintenance of normal serum albumin levels in the early postoperative period when capillary beds appear to be more permeable, and decrease in osmotic pressure of the plasma may be more catastrophic. Maintenance of adequate total caloric intake and balance of alimentation should be the long-term goal.

REFERENCES

2-1.   Stare, F. J.: Nutrition in medicine. Bull. N.Y. Acad. Med. 20:237, 1944.

2-2.   Brozek, J.: Body composition. The relative amounts of fat, tissue, and water vary with age, sex, exercise, and nutritional state. Science 134:920, 1961.

2-3.   Cahill, G. F., Jr.: Body fuels and their metabolism. Bull. Am. Coll. Surgeons, November 1970, p. 12.

2-4.   Cahill, G. F., Jr.: Starvation in man. New Engl. J. Med. 282:668, 1970.

2-5.   Winitz, M., Graff, J., Gallagher, V., Narkin, A., and Seedman, D. A.: Evaluation of chemical diets as nutrition for man-in-space. Nature 205:741, 1965.

2-6.   Dudrick, S. J., Wilmore, D. W., Vars, H. M., and Rhoads, J. E.: Can intravenous feeding as the sole means of nutrition support growth in the child and restore weight loss in an adult? An affirmative answer. Ann. Surg. 169:974, 1969.

2-7.   Levenson, S. M., Birkhill, F. R., and Waterman, D. F.: The healing of soft tissue wounds: the effects of nutrition, anemia, and age. Surgery 28:905, 1950.

2-8.   Guyton, A. C., and Lindsey, A. W: Effect of elevated left atrial pressure and decreased plasma protein concentration on the development of pulmonary edema. Circ. Res. 7:649, 1959.

2-9.   English, T. A. H., Digerness, S. B., Kirklin, J. W., and Karp, R. B.: Pulmonary capillary blood volume and lung water in pulmonary edema. Surg. Gynec. Obst. 132:93, 1971.

2-10. Clark, A. H.: The effect of diet on the healing of wounds. Bull. Johns Hopkins Hosp. 30:117, 1919.

2-11. Thompson, W. D., Ravdin, I. S., and Frank, I. L.: Effect of hypoproteinemia on wound disruption. Arch. Surg. 36:500, 1938.

2-12. Marsh, R. L., Coxe, J. W., III., Ross, W. L., and Stevens, G. A.: Factors involving wound dehiscence. Study of one thousand cases. JAMA 155:1197, 1954.

2-13. Localio, S. A., Chassin, J. L., and Hinton, J. W.: Tissue protein depletion. A factor in wound disruption. Surg. Gynec. Obst. 86:107, 1948.

2-14. Localio, S. A., Morgan, M. E., and Hinton, J. W.: The biological chemistry of wound healing. I. The effect of dl-methionine on the healing of wounds in protein-depleted animals. Surg. Gynec. Obst. 86:582, 1948.

2-15. Caldwell, F. T., Jr., Rosenberg, I. K., Rosenberg, B. F., and Mishra, O. P.: Effect of single amino acid supplementation upon the gain of tensile strength of wounds in protein-depleted rats. Surg. Gynec. Obst. 119:823, 1964.

2-16. Rosenthal, S., Lerner, B., DiBiase, F., and Enquist, I. F.: Relation of strength to composition in diabetic wounds. Surg. Gynec. Obst. 115:437, 1962.

2-17. Howard, J. M., Barker, W. F., Culbertson, W. R., Grotzinger, P. J., Iovine, V. M., Keehn, R. J., and Ravdin, R. G. (eds.): Postoperative wound infections: The influence of ultraviolet irradiation of the operating room and of various other factors. Ann. Surg. 160: (Supplement with No. 2) 56, 1964.

2-18. Benedict, F. G.: A study of prolonged fasting. Washington, D.C., Carnegie Institute, 1915, Publication No. 203.

2-19. Stephens, R. V., and Randall, H. T.: Use of a concentrated, balanced, liquid elemental diet for nutritional management in catabolic states. Ann. Surg. 170:642, 1969.

2-20. Owen, O. E., Felig, P., Morgan, A. P., Wahren, J., and Cahill, G. F., Jr.: Liver and kidney metabolism during prolonged starvation. J. Clin. Invest. 48:574, 1969.

2-21. Marliss, E. B., Aoki, T. T., Unger, R. H., Soeldner, J. S., and Cahill, G. F., Jr.: Glucagon levels and metabolic effects in fasting man. J. Clin. Invest. 49:2256, 1970.

2-22. Gump, F. E., Kinney, J. M., and Price, J. B., Jr.: Energy metabolism in surgical patients: Oxygen consumption and blood flow. J. Surg. Res. 10:613, 1970.

2-23. Cuthbertson, D. P.: CXXXVII. The disturbance of metabolism produced by bony and non-bony injury, with notes on certain abnormal conditions of bone. Biochem. J. 24:1244, 1930.

2-24. Moore, F. D.: Bodily changes in surgical convalescence. I. The normal sequence—observations and interpretations. Ann. Surg. 137:289, 1953.

2-25. Fleck, A., and Munro, H. N.: Protein metabolism after injury. Metabolism 12:783, 1963.

2-26. Moore, F. D.: Editorial. The significance of weight changes after trauma. Ann. Surg. 141:141, 1955.

2-27. Pareira, M. D., Conrad, E. J., Hicks, W., and Elman, R.: Therapeutic nutrition with tube feeding. JAMA 156:810, 1954.

2-28. Rush, B. F., Jr., Richardson, J. D., and Griffen, W. O., Jr.: Positive nitrogen balance immediately after abdominal operations. Am. J. Surg. 119:70, 1970.

2-29. Johnston, I. D. A., Marino, J. D., and Stevens, J. Z.: The effect of intravenous feeding on the balances of nitrogen, sodium, and potassium after operation. Brit. J. Surg. 53:885, 1966.

2-30. Warner, W. A.: Release of free fatty acids following trauma. J. Trauma 9:602, 1969.

2-31. Mays, E. T.: The effect of surgical stress of plasma free fatty acids. J. Surg. Res. 10:315, 1970.

2-32. Bridges, J. M., Dalby, A. M., Hadden, D. R., Johnston, H. A., and Weaver, J. A.: The effect of "in-vivo" alteration of free fatty acids on platelet stickiness. J. Atheroscler. Res. 7:695, 1967.

2-33. Hoak, J. C., Poole, J. C. F., and Robinson, D. S.: Thrombosis associated with mobilization of fatty acids. Am. J. Path. 43:987, 1963.

2-34. Kinney, J. M., Long, C. L., Gump, F. E., and Duke, J. H., Jr.: Tissue composition of weight loss in surgical patients. I. Elective operation. Ann. Surg. 168:459, 1968.

2-35. Im, M. J. C., and Hoopes, J. E.: Energy metabolism in healing skin wounds. J. Surg. Res. 10:459, 1970.

2-36. Kinney, J. M., and Roe, F.: Caloric equivalent of fever: I. Patterns of postoperative response. Ann. Surg. 156:610, 1962.

2-37. DuBois, E. F.: Basal Metabolism in Health and Disease. 2nd ed. Philadelphia, Lea & Febiger, 1927.

2-38. Roe, C. F., and Kinney, J. M.: The caloric equivalent of fever: II. Influence of major trauma. Ann. Surg. 161:140, 1965.

2-39. Roe, C. F., Kinney, J. M., and Blair, C.: Water and heat exchange in third-degree burns. Surgery 56:212, 1964.

2-40. Jelenko, C., III., Wheeler, M. L., and Anderson, A. P.: The effect of topical sulfamylon on water loss through burn eschar: a re-evaluation. J. Trauma 10:1123, 1970.

2-41. Moser, M. H., Robinson, D. W., and Schloerb, P. R.: Transfers of water and electrolytes across granulation tissue in patients following burns. Surg. Gynec. Obst. 118:984, 1964.

2-42. Harrison, H. N., Moncrief, J. A., Duckett, J. W., Jr., and Mason, A. D., Jr: The relationship between energy metabolism and water loss from vaporization in severely burned patients. Surgery 56: 203, 1964.

2-43. Munster, A. M., Hoagland, H. C., and Pruitt, B. A., Jr.: The effect of thermal injury on serum immunoglobulins. Ann. Surg. 172: 965, 1970.

2-44. Thomsen, V.: Studies of trauma and carbohydrate metabolism with special reference to the existence of traumatic diabetes. Acta Med. Scand. Suppl. 91, 1:416, 1938.

2-45. Hayes, M. A., and Brandt, R. L.: Carbohydrate metabolism in the immediate postoperative period. Surgery 32:819, 1952.

2-46. Schumer, W.: Metabolic considerations in the preoperative evaluation of the surgical patient. Surg. Gynec. Obst. 121:611, 1965.

2-47. Porte, D., Jr. and Bierman, E. L.: A new, nonisotopic method for the measurement of triglyceride turnover rate in man. (abstr.) J. Clin. Invest. 46:1105, 1967.

2-48. Borgstrom, B., Dahlqvist, A., Lundh, G., and Sjovall, J.: Studies of intestinal digestion and absorption in the human. J. Clin. Invest. 36:1251, 1957.

2-49. Shingleton, W. W., Baylin, G. J., Isley, J. K., Sanders, A. P., and Ruffin, J. M.: A study of fat absorption after gastric surgery using I^{131}-labeled fat. Ann. Surg. 144:433, 1956.

2-50. Riklis, E., and Quastel, J. H.: Effects of cations on sugar absorption by isolated surviving guinea pig intestine. Canad. J. Biochem. Phys. 36:347, 1958.

2-51. Curran, P. F.: Ion transport in intestine and its coupling to other transport processes. Fed. Proc. 24:993, 1965.

2-52. Gardner, J. D., Brown, M. S., and Laster, L.: The columnar epithelial cell of the small intestine: Digestion and transport. New Engl. J. Med. 283:1196, 1970.

2-53. Jordan, P. H., Jr.: Physiology of the small intestine. Surg. Gynec. Obst. 124:1331, 1967.

2-54. Hofmann, A. F.: A physicochemical approach to the intraluminal phase of fat absorption. Gastroenterology 50:56, 1966.

2-55. Heaton, K. W., Austad, W. I., Lack, L., and Tyor, M. P.: Entero-hepatic circulation of C^{14}-labeled bile salts in disorders of the distal small bowel. Gastroenterology 55:5, 1968.

2-56. Alpers, D., Wessler, S., and Avioli, L. V.: Ileal resection and bile salt metabolism. JAMA 215:101, 1971.

2-57. Sun, D. C. H., Albacete, R. A., and Chen, J. K.: Malabsorption studies in cirrhosis of the liver. Arch. Intern. Med. 119:567, 1967.

2-58. Welch, C. E.: Abdominal surgery (second of three parts). New Engl. J. Med. 284:471, 1971.

2-59. Winawer, S. J., Broitman, S. A., Wolochow, D. A., Osborne, M. P., and Zamcheck, N.: Successful management of massive small-bowel resection based on assessment of absorption defects and nutritional need. New Engl. J. Med. 274:72, 1966.

2-60. Bothe, F. A., Magee, W. S., and Driscoll, R. H.: A massive resection of small intestine from fifteen centimeters distal to the ligament of Treitz to within six centimeters of the ileocecal valve—with a four year follow-up. Ann. Surg. 140:755, 1954.

2-61. Booth, C. C.: The Metabolic Effects of Intestinal Resection in Man. Postgrad. Med. J. 37:725, 1961.

2-62. LeVeen, H. H., Borek, B., Axelrod, D. B., and Johnson, A.: Cause and treatment of diarrhea following resection of the small intestine. Surg. Gynec. Obst. 124:766, 1967.

2-63. Osborne, M. P., Sizer, J., Frederick, P. L., and Zamcheck, N.: Massive bowel resection and gastric hypersecretion. Its mechanism and a plan for clinical study and management. Am. J. Surg. 114:393, 1967.

2-64. Flint, J. M.: The effect of extensive resections of the small intestine. Bull. Johns Hopkins Hosp. 23:127, 1912.

2-65. Loran, M. R., and Althausen, T. L.: Cellular proliferation of intestinal epithelia in the rat two months after partial resection of the ileum. J. Biophys. and Biochem. Cytol. 7:667, 1960.

2-66. Wright, H. K., and Titson, M. D.: The short gut syndrome—pathophysiology and treatment. Curr. Prob. Surg., June 1971.

2-67. Levitan, R.: Colonic absorption of electrolytes and water. Am. J. Clin. Nutr. 22:315, 1969.

2-68. Gorbach, S. L.: Intestinal microflora. Gastroenterology 60:1110, 1971.

2-69. Kalser, M. H., Cohen, R., Arteaga, I., Yawn, E., Mayoral, L., Hoffert, W. R., and Frazier, D.: Normal viral and bacterial flora of the human small and large intestine. New Engl. J. Med. 174:500, 1966.

2-70. Kalser, M. H., Cohen, R., Arteaga, I., Yawn, E., Mayoral, L., Hoffert, W., and Frazier, D.: Normal viral and bacterial flora of the human small and large intestine (concluded). New Engl. J. Med. 274:558, 1966.

2-71. Cohen, R., Roth, F. J., Delgado, E., Ahearn, D. G., and Kalser, M. H.: Fungal flora of the normal human small and large intestine. New Engl. J. Med. 280:638, 1969.

2-72. Donaldson, R. M., Jr.: Normal bacterial populations of the intestine and their relation to intestinal function. New Engl. J. Med. 270: 938, 1964.

2-73. Blacklock, J. W. S., Guthrie, K. J., and Macpherson, I.: A study of the intestinal flora of children. J. Path. Bact. 44:321, 1937.

2-74. Zeldow, B. J.: Studies on the antibacterial action of human saliva. II. Observations on the mode of action of a lactobacillus bactericidin. J. Dent. Res. 40:446, 1961.

2-75. Williams, N. B., and Powlen, D. O.: Human parotid saliva as a sole source of nutrient for micro-organisms. Arch. Oral Biol. 1:48, 1959.

2-76. Wirts, C. W., and Goldstein, F.: Studies of the mechanism of postgastrectomy steatorrhea. Ann. Intern. Med. 58:25, 1963.

2-77. Dixon, J. M. S.: The fate of bacteria in the small intestine. J. Path. Bact. 79:131, 1960.

2-78. Brown, H., and McDermott, W. V., Jr.: Current management of post-shunt hepatic encephalopathy. Presented at the annual meeting of the New England Surgical Society, Mountain View House, Oct. 20, 1967.

2-79. Rosenberg, I. H., Hardison, W. G., and Bull, D. M.: Abnormal bile-salt patterns and intestinal bacterial overgrowth associated with malabsorption. New Engl. J. Med. 276:1391, 1967.

2-80. Ragins, H., and Oberhelman, H. A., Jr.: Anemia associated with a stagnant ("blind") jejunal loop. Arch. Surg. 80:524, 1960.

2-81. Ainley, N. J., and Lamb, D. C.: Megaloblastic anemia following operations on the small intestine. Brit. J. Surg. 608, 1959.

2-82. Floch, M. H.: Recent contributions in intestinal absorption and malabsorption. Am. J. Clin. Nutr. 22:327, 1969.

2-83. Smith, M. K., Jepson, R. P., and Catchpole, B. N.: Ileus: An experimental study. Brit. J. Surg. 52:381, 1965.

2-84. Handley, W. S.: Paralytic ileus in acute appendicitis. Lancet 2:1120, 1935.

2-85. Burn, J. H.: A new view of adrenergic nerve fibres, explaining the action of reserpine, bretylium, and guanethidine. Brit. Med. J. 1:1623, 1961.

2-86. Samuel, E.: Some mechanical syndromes following partial gastrectomy. J. Royal Coll. Surg., Edin. 6:179, 1961.

2-87. Wells, C., Tinckler, L., Rawlinson, K., Jones, H., and Saunders, J.: Postoperative gastrointestinal motility. Lancet 1:4, 1964.

2-88. Rothnie, N. G., Harper, R. A. K., and Catchpole, B. N.: Early postoperative gastrointestinal activity. Lancet 2:64, 1963.

2-89. Wells, C., Rawlinson, K., Tinckler, L., Jones, H., and Saunders, J.: Ileus and postoperative intestinal motility. Lancet 2:136, 1961.

2-90. Glucksman, D. L., Kalser, M. H., and Warren, W. D.: Small intestinal absorption in the immediate postoperative period. Surgery 60: 1020, 1966.

2-91. Levitt, M. D.: Volume and composition of human intestinal gas determined by means of an intestinal washout technic. New Engl. J. Med. 284:1394, 1971.

2-92. Wright, H. K., O'Brien, J. J., and Tilson, M. D.: Water absorption in experimental closed segment obstruction of the ileum in man. Am. J. Surg. 121:96, 1971.

2-93. Anderson, R. E., Schmidtke, W. H., and Diffenbaugh, W. G.: Influence of an increased intraluminal pressure on intestinal absorption. Ann. Surg. 156:276, 1962.

2-94. van de Kamer, J. H., ten Bokkel Huinink, H., and Weyers, H. A.: Rapid method for the determination of fat in feces. J. Biol. Chem. 177:347, 1949.

2-95. Ingelfinger, F. J.: For want of an enzyme. Nutr. Today 3:2, 1968.

2-96. Sleisenger, M. H.: Malabsorption syndrome. New Engl. J. Med. 281:1111, 1969.

2-97. Whipple, G. H.: Hemoglobin and plasma proteins: Their production, utilization and interrelation. Am. J. Med. Sci. 203:477, 1942.

2-98. Allen, J. G., Stemmer, E., and Head, L. R.: Similar growth rates of litter mate puppies maintained on oral protein with those on the same quantity of protein as daily intravenous plasma for 99 days as only protein source. Ann. Surg. 144:349, 1956.

2-99. Rice, C. O., Orr, B., and Enquist, I.: Parenteral nutrition in the surgical patient as provided from glucose, amino acids and alcohol. Ann. Surg. 131:289, 1950.

2-100. Holt, L. E., Jr., Tidwell, H. C., and Scott, T. F. McN.: The intravenous administration of fat. A practical therapeutic procedure. J. Pediat. 6:151, 1935.

2-101. Jordan, P. H., Jr., Wilson, P., and Stuart, J.: Observations on patient tolerance with intravenous administration of fat emulsion. Surg. Gynec. Obst. 102:737, 1956.

2-102. Dudrick, S. J., Rhoads, J. E., and Vars, H. M. Growth of puppies receiving all nutritional requirements by vein. Fortschr. Parenteral Ernahrung 2:16, 1967.

2-103. Dudrick, S. J., Wilmore, D. W., and Vars, H. M.: Long-term total parenteral nutrition with growth in puppies and positive nitrogen balance in patients. Surg. Forum 18:356, 1967.

2-104. Wilmore, D. W., and Dudrick, S. J.: Growth and development of an infant receiving all nutrients exclusively by vein. JAMA 203: 860, 1968.

2-105. Dudrick, S. J., Wilmore, D. W., Steiger, E., Mackie, J. A., and Fitts,

W. T., Jr.: Spontaneous closure of traumatic pancreatoduodenal fistulas with total intravenous nutrition. J. Trauma 10:542, 1970.

2-106. Dudrick, S. J., Steiger, E., and Long, J. M.: Renal failure in surgical patients. Treatment with intravenous essential amino acids and hypertonic glucose. Surgery 68:180, 1970.

2-107. Filler, R. M., Eraklis, A. J., Rubin, V. G., and Das, J. B.: Long-term total parenteral nutrition in infants. New Engl. J. Med. 281:589, 1969.

2-108. Rea, W. J., Wyrick, W. J., Jr., McClelland, R. N., and Webb, W. R.: Intravenous hyperosmolar alimentation. Arch. Surg. 100:393, 1970.

2-109. Shils, M. E., Wright, W. L., Turnbull, A., and Brescia, F.: Long-term parenteral nutrition through an external arteriovenous shunt. New Engl. J. Med. 283:341, 1970.

2-110. Scribner, B. H., Cole, J. J., Christopher, T. G., Vizzo, J. E., Atkins, R. C., and Blagg, C. R.: Long-term total parenteral nutrition. The concept of an artificial gut. JAMA 212:457, 1970.

3

KIDNEY

PRIMARY FUNCTION

The function of the kidney is to regulate body-water volume, to regulate the concentration of electrolytes in the body fluids, and to eliminate certain products of body metabolism. Renal function provides the only mechanism for elimination of the nitrogen released by the metabolism of protein, and failure of the kidney is heralded by an increase in the level of nitrogenous compounds in the blood. In addition to regulating the concentrations of all electrolytes, the kidney, through its control of sodium excretion, regulates the extracellular fluid volume, and indirectly the volume of intracellular water.

GENERAL ANATOMY AND PHYSIOLOGY

The kidney is a tense, turgid organ containing billions of nephron units whose glomeruli and tubules lie in a dynamic interstitial fluid space. Cortical nephron units are perfused by a large amount of rapidly moving blood, and vasoactivity is directly related to the regulation of glomerular perfusion. Juxtamedullary glomeruli are perfused by the inner cortical blood flow, a portion of which is directed into the vasae rectae leading to the tip of the medullary tuft. In the medulla, blood flow is slower. Here concentration and dilution take place, and vasomotion may be independent of glomerular perfusion. Interstitial pressure appears to be regulated by both pressure and resistance factors in the arterioles and by the concentration of osmotically active solute in the interstitial fluid. Changes in pressure and interstitial fluid osmolality affect the functioning of tubular cells [3-1].

Vascular System

The kidney is uniquely designed to perform its function. The large flow of renal blood, far larger than that necessary for nutrition of the renal parenchyma, enters through the renal arterial system. Primary interlobar branches of the renal artery reach between each papillary protrusion of the medulla to divide at the level of the corticomedullary junction into an arcuate system, arching transversely between the cortex and the medulla. From these arcuate vessels interlobular arteries reach into the cortex to supply the glomerular tufts. Efferent arterioles lead from the glomerular capillaries to supply the interstitial capillary network in the medulla and cortex, and in the medulla, to become vasae rectae, reaching down to the papillary tip. Interlobular renal veins drain the interstitial tissue and recapitulate the arterial circulation by joining together to form arcuate veins, interlobar veins, and the main renal venous system [3-2].

Blood-Flow Dynamics

Blood flow to the kidney has been studied by a variety of indicator techniques using xenon 133, krypton 85, rubidium 86, and potassium 42 [3-3, 3-4, 3-5]. All studies show that 80 to 85 per cent of renal blood flow rapidly traverses the cortex while approximately 11 per cent flows more slowly through the outer medulla and inner cortical area. Two to 3 per cent flows through the medulla and papillae and this small amount proceeds at a much slower rate.

Renal-Tissue Tension

The vascular configuration—namely the entry of arterial blood through a hilar pedicle, the distribution of blood throughout the renal parenchyma, and its exit through hilar veins—allows a specific tissue tension or turgor to be produced in the kidney dependent upon arterial blood pressure and outflow resistance. This tissue tension may play an important role in regulating the excretion of sodium. The functional distention of the kidney produced by arterial inflow has been studied by Swann, who has shown that under normal conditions one-third of the volume of the functioning kidney consists of fluid, maintained in the vascular system and the interstitium by arterial pressure. This tension is maintained at physiologic levels by functional obstruction to venous outflow which occurs at the junction of interlobar and arcuate veins [3-6, 3-7].

Functional Zones

The human kidney appears to have several distinct functional zones. The main portion of the cortex is occupied by glomeruli which have relatively short tubule systems. These tubules lie almost entirely within the cortex and are surrounded by capillary networks. They empty into collecting ducts which run from the cortex to the papillary tip. Approximately 85 per cent of functioning glomeruli lie within this cortical zone. In the inner cortex lie the juxtamedullary glomeruli, approximately 15 per cent of the total. These glomeruli differ from the outer cortical glomeruli in that the tubular systems reach deep into the medulla, forming long loops. The efferent arterioles of these glomeruli do not break up to form an immediate capillary bed. They are muscular arterioles which run in long loops, parallel to the long loops of the tubules. It is the function of these loops and the vasae rectae to regulate medullary concentration of solute via the countercurrent multiplier and exchanger mechanism.

The collecting ducts, which contain postloop filtrate from all glomeruli, traverse the medullary tissue on their way to the renal pelvis. In this passage final urinary concentration is achieved by regulation of water resorption. Thus the action of the tubules and vasae rectae of the juxtamedullary glomeruli controls the final concentration of the urine, through water excretion and resorption.

Nerve Supply

The sympathetic innervation of the kidney plays an important role in the renal response to alterations in blood pressure and cardiac output. Adrenergic innervation has been shown by histochemical studies in the interlobar, arcuate, and interlobular arteries and along the afferent arterioles. These fibers also are present in the vasae rectae of the outer medulla [3-8]. The importance of adrenergic control of medullary arterioles which supply the juxtamedullary glomeruli and continue as the vasae rectae has been pointed out by Ljungqvist and Wagermark [3-9]. Their studies show that cortical blood flow must traverse the glomerular tuft, whereas juxtamedullary blood flow and medullary blood flow may bypass the glomerulus. Increase in sympathetic activity results in a rise in afferent arteriolar resistance, with a fall in glomerular filtration. Interstitial pressure falls, accompanied by an increase in sodium resorption. Increased tone in the muscular vasae rectae reduces medullary blood flow, slows the flow in the countercurrent system, and permits increased medullary concentration.

NORMAL RENAL FUNCTION

Glomerular Filtration

The excretory function of the kidney depends on adequate filtration of plasma. The rate of filtration by the glomeruli can be measured by the use of substances which are filtered and neither resorbed nor excreted by tubular cells. By means of injected inulin or by the measurement of naturally occurring creatinine, clearance studies can be performed indicating the glomerular filtration rate (GFR). In normal adult man, the GFR ranges from 100 to 120 ml/min [3-10, 3-11, 3-12]. The glomerular filtration rate normally falls with increasing age, presumably due to changes in renal vasculature [3-13, 3-14].

Under basal metabolic conditions a glomerular filtration rate of approximately 30 ml/min will filter enough plasma to maintain normal body composition. A decrease below this level results in the accumulation of nitrogen-containing compounds within the blood. The presence of a normal BUN or blood creatinine, therefore, indicates only that renal function is at or above this minimal level—i.e., that glomerular filtration rate is at least 30 ml/min. These blood studies do not indicate renal reserve nor show the actual level of filtration or the number of functioning nephron units.

Inadequate filtration also prevents proper excretion of certain other ions, namely potassium and phosphorus. A rise in serum potassium occurs, the rate of rise depending on the amount of potassium liberated from endogenous protein, which in turn is dependent upon energy needs and administered fuel substances. Potassium levels may rise rapidly when tissue damage is present.

Hyperphosphatemia also occurs when filtration is inadequate. In chronic states this causes hypocalcemia, which in turn results in stimulation of secretion of parathyroid hormone (secondary hyperparathyroidism [3-15].

Proximal Tubular Function

Adequate function of tubular cells is necessary for the regulation of electrolytes and water. Under normal conditions, almost all of the glomerular filtrate is resorbed in the tubule. Thus, of a total of approximately 140 liters filtered each 24 hr, usually only 1 to 2 liters of urine are excreted. Most of this resorption occurs isotonically in the proximal tubule.

Proximal tubular resorption returns most of the water and contained small ions to the blood. All filtered potassium is resorbed here. Calcium [3-16], magnesium [3-17], and phosphorus [3-18] are resorbed in amounts from 95 to 99 per cent of the filtered load. Sodium and bicarbonate are isotonically resorbed, the amount resorbed depending upon the dynamics of the extracellular fluid.

EFFECTS OF CHANGE IN EXTRACELLULAR FLUID VOLUME

Proximal tubular resorption is most directly influenced by the adequacy of extracellular fluid volume. Expansion of the extracellular space causes a decrease in proximal sodium and water resorption with increase in excretion [3-19]. This appears to be due to local changes within the renal parenchyma and tubular cells [3-20, 3-21]. Vascular factors seem to play an important role in proximal sodium regulation. Increased blood flow due to elevation of cardiac output or to local vasodilatation causes naturesis [3-22], as does the elevation of perfusion pressure [3-23, 3-24]. Changes in cardiac output due to volume expansion have been shown to increase renal interstitial pressure [3-25] and such increase in tissue pressure may in itself inhibit resorption of sodium in the proximal tubule [3-26, 3-27, 3-28].

NEURAL CONTROL

The importance of normal vasomotor control of the kidney in the proper regulation of sodium excretion has been clearly shown in man, and blockade of normal adrenergic vasomotion results in an inability to properly conserve sodium [3-29, 3-30].

EFFECTS DUE TO CHANGES IN HEMATOCRIT AND PLASMA

Plasma and interstitial composition also plays an important role in regulation of sodium excretion, and proximal sodium resorption is enhanced by elevation of the plasma oncotic pressure [3-31]. Changes in hematocrit can also influence renal hemodynamics and sodium resorption. A decrease in hematocrit increases renal plasma flow and decreases renal vascular resistance [3-32]. Accompanying this change is an increase in sodium and potassium excretion [3-33].

DIURETICS

The diuretics most often used in surgical patients have their major effect on proximal tubular resorption of ions and water. Mannitol acts as an osmotic diuretic. The mannitol molecule must be filtered and must appear in the proximal tubular fluid for diuresis to occur. This molecule cannot be removed from the fluid by tubular resorption. To satisfy isotonicity, water is held in the tubule, with a net decrease in tubular resorption and increase in excreted urine volume.

Ethacrynic acid and furosemide act to block proximal tubular resorption of sodium and thus to prevent resorption of the associated water. The mechanism is as yet not well understood. The result is the excretion of up to 25 per cent of the filtered sodium with large volumes of water. Also excreted are large amounts of calcium and magnesium due to this proximal tubular action. These diuretics provide the most effective means of rapidly reducing serum calcium levels in hypercalcemic states [3-34].

Distal Tubular Function

Distal tubular cell function provides the mechanism for excretion or resorption of electrolyte-free water; for excretion of specific ions, especially potassium, and for the regulation of acid-base balance by hydrogen or bicarbonate ion excretion.

CONTROL OF WATER EXCRETION

Regulation of water excretion by the distal tubule and collecting duct of the nephron is the main mechanism for maintenance of normal serum osmolality. The excretion of free water (C_{H_2O}) is accomplished by pumping sodium from the tubule into the interstitium in the ascending Loop of Henle and collecting duct. In the absence of antidiuretic hormone, tubular cells in these areas are impermeable to water. Therefore, removal of sodium ion decreases tubular fluid concentration below the concentration of the serum. The hypotonic tubular fluid then contains some electrolyte-free water which can proceed through the collecting duct and be excreted. Excretion of free water thus depends on the delivery of an adequate amount of sodium to the distal tubule and the availability of normal aerobic metabolism in the tubular cells [3-35, 3-36].

Antidiuretic Hormone. The secretion of antidiuretic hormone must be inhibited to maintain the tubular cells in the water-impermeable state. Verney showed in 1947 that inhibition could be caused by the administration of a water load, and that it was mediated via osmoreceptors in the hypothalamus [3-37]. This state of "physiologic diabetes insipidus" occurred in response to a decrease in serum osmolality. Inhibition of antidiuretic hormone secretion is also produced by elevation of blood alcohol levels. [3-38].

Increase in the permeability of tubular cells to water is produced by the presence of antidiuretic hormone. Resorption of free water (T_{CH_2O}) to increase urinary concentration is an energy-requiring mechanism. Adequate amounts of sodium must be present in the distal tubule to allow free water resorption, since water moves only with the sodium ion from the tubule to the interstitium.

Control of Antidiuretic Hormone Secretion. In man and many other mammals the balance of renal feedback mechanisms is designed to protect body-fluid volume. Thus there are only two major stimuli that inhibit the production of antidiuretic hormone: decrease in serum osmolality, and rise in blood-alcohol levels. However, there are many stimuli that cause secretion of antidiuretic hormone (ADH), resulting in interruption of water diuresis, expansion of fluid volume, and decrease in serum tonicity. Verney noted in his original experiments that interruption of diuresis occurred due to emotional disturbances [3-37]. He also documented the stimulation of ADH secretion by hypertonic perfusion of the hypothalamus.

It has been shown that hypovolemia of 10 per cent of blood volume stimulates ADH secretion due to activation of atrial receptors, while blood loss of larger amounts produces a further increase in secretory rate through activation of aortic baroreceptors [3-39]. Arterial baroreceptor activity appears to be responsive to pulse pressure in the aorta and carotid arteries [3-40]. The sensitivity of the intrathoracic venous receptors can be shown by the demonstration that ADH levels decrease in the supine position, and rise moderately in the standing position. In addition, exposure to cold with diversion of blood from skin to central core circulation reduces ADH levels whereas exposure to a warm atmosphere allows ADH levels to rise [3-41].

Antidiuretic Hormone Secretion After Trauma. Studies by Moran et al have shown that surgical operation and trauma produce maximal increases in ADH levels beginning with the trauma of skin incision and lasting over a four to five day posttrauma period [3-42]. These studies explain the susceptibility of the postsurgical or posttraumatic patient to water retention and hypotonicity. Such changes are absent in patients with ADH lack due to diabetes insipidus [3-43, 3-44].

Metabolism of Antidiuretic Hormone. The action of ADH is of short duration. The vasoconstriction caused by local injection into an artery disappears within three minutes after cessation of infusion. The diuretic renal response noted by Verney requires 10 to 15 min to occur after cessation of vasopressin infusion. Clearance of vasopressin from the circulation is performed by the removal of a constant fraction of the existing level by liver and kidney. Thus patients with liver disease show a prolonged time of action of vasopressin [3-45].

CONTROL OF SODIUM EXCRETION

Sodium resorption by the distal tubule may be directly affected by expansion of the circulating volume, with decrease in absorption occurring during volume expansion [3-46].

Aldosterone. The major influence on sodium resorption in the distal tubule is the adrenal cortical hormone, aldosterone [3-47, 3-48]. This substance was detected in adrenal tissue by Grundy et al in 1951 [3-49]. Many physiologic studies since that time have confirmed its primary activity on sodium resorption in the distal tubule. Absence of aldosterone in patients with adrenal insufficiency produces sodium loss, hyponatremia, shock, and death. Hyperaldosteronism produced by hyperfunctioning adenoma, or by adrenal cortical hyperplasia, causes sodium retention, potassium loss, overexpansion of the extracellular fluid, and hypertension.

Control of Aldosterone Secretion. Release of aldosterone from the zona glomerulosa cells of the adrenal is mediated by the release of renin from the juxtaglomerular cells surrounding the afferent arteriole of the kidney; the conversion of renin to angiotensin I and II; and the direct stimulation of aldosterone release of angiotensin II [3-50, 3-51, 3-52]. Increase in renal renin secretion and thus increase in aldosterone secretion, has been shown to occur following reduction in perfusion pressure of the kidney, decrease in circulating blood volume, and in states of acute and chronic sodium depletion [3-53, 3-54]. The exact stimulus for renin release from the juxtaglomerular apparatus under such conditions is not known, but alteration in renal tissue pressure has been suggested [3-55], as has change in distal tubular sodium concentration [3-56]. Possibly both factors are at work. Normal innervation appears to be necessary for appropriate renin release to occur [3-57].

CONTROL OF EXCRETION OF OTHER IONS

The distal renal tubule is the site of regulation of hydrogen, bicarbonate, and potassium excretion. The resorption of excretion of these ions by the distal tubule is related to the amount of sodium in the tubular fluid and to the rate at which sodium is resorbed—regulated in great part by aldosterone.

Potassium. Glomerular filtration places the plasma filtrate in the tubule. From this filtrate all of the potassium and a large portion of the bicarbonate ion are resorbed in the proximal tubule. Potassium excretion, therefore, occurs by exchange of potassium into the tubule and sodium out of the tubule in the distal segment.

Bicarbonate. Bicarbonate excretion occurs when distal tubular bicarbonate is not completely resorbed. It is now known that the bulk of bicarbonate resorption occurs through a mechanism of hydrogen-ion secretion. Filtered bicarbonate combines with secreted hydrogen ion to form carbonic acid. The latter is then dehydrated to carbon dioxide which diffuses out of the lumen. The presence of carbonic anhydrase at the luminal membrane of the proximal tubule is required for prompt dehydration of carbonic acid.

Hydrogen. Hydrogen-ion excretion occurs by three mechanisms: first, the complete absorption of all bicarbonate; second, the acidification of ammonia to ammonium, and excretion of the latter in the urine; third, the creation of titratable acid by the acidification of hyposulfate and hypophosphate. The change of monohydrogen phosphate to dihydrogen phosphate eliminates one hydrogen ion, and the same occurs when diffusable base ammonia reaches tubular fluid and accepts one hydrogen ion to form the nondiffusable ammonium ion.

IMPORTANCE OF SODIUM ION

Metabolism of fuel substrates creates a load of metabolic acid, potassium, and nitrogen which must be excreted to prevent the occurrence of acidosis and hyperkalemia. Inasmuch as hydrogen, sodium, and potassium exchange must be balanced to maintain electroneutrality, distal resorption of large amounts of sodium will require excretion of similarly

large amounts of potassium and hydrogen ion, and the formation of
an acid urine. Similarly, rejection of sodium by the distal tubule will
prevent hydrogen-ion excretion and will allow the formation of an alkaline urine [3-58]. It is clear that an insufficient amount of sodium
ion in the distal tubule due to decrease in filtration rate will prevent
the excretion of hydrogen and potassium ion [3-59].

Excretion of Acids

Acid excretion by the kidney responds to an increase in acidity
of body fluids whether from respiratory or metabolic change. In states
of chronic acidosis, an increase in hydrogen excretion is accomplished
by an increase in the conversion of ammonia to ammonium. This change
is in response to an increase in the breakdown of glutamine. Increased
glutaminase enzymes are found in the kidney in such conditions [3-60].

EFFECT OF SODIUM CHLORIDE

The presence of an absorbable anion such as chloride in the distal
tubule allows resorption of sodium chloride without the necessity for
excretion of hydrogen, whereas the presence of a nonabsorbable anion
such as hypophosphate allows an exchange of hydrogen for sodium. Administration of sodium chloride solutions thus may aggravate acidosis,
while solutions with less chloride than sodium (Ringer's lactate) allow
hydrogen-ion excretion. Decrease in extracellular fluid inhibits this entire mechanism because less sodium is present in the distal tubule.

Excretion of Alkali

The renal correction of metabolic alkalosis with an increase in
body bicarbonate requires the excretion of bicarbonate ion. Metabolic
alkalosis of the usual type, due to excess vomiting of acid stomach contents, is associated with normal levels of plasma sodium and depressed
levels of plasma chloride.

IMPORTANCE OF PLASMA SODIUM-CHLORIDE GAP

Until chloride levels are corrected, alkalosis may be difficult to correct due to the sodium exchange mechanism. The sodium which matches
nonabsorbable anions (nonchloride anions) must be exchanged for hydrogen or potassium which are then excreted. The sodium which matches

chloride may be resorbed without such exchange. If a large difference between sodium and chloride levels exists, increased hydrogen and/or potassium excretion will occur and bicarbonate excretion will be impossible. Therefore, the therapy of metabolic alkalosis must include restoration of chloride levels to normal. Potassium stores are usually depleted in this state in an attempt to use potassium as an exchange for sodium rather than hydrogen. Schwartz has shown, however, that restoration of potassium stores is not required to correct the alkalosis [3-61].

Effects of Electrolyte Imbalance on Renal Function

POTASSIUM DEPLETION

Changes in serum electrolytes affect the function of the kidney. Potassium depletion produces an inability to concentrate the urine normally while the diluting ability may remain unimpaired. Excretion of a large sodium load is impaired, as is the ability of the kidney to reduce sodium excretion to low rates. Although it was originally thought that bicarbonate excretion could not be accomplished under conditions of potassium depletion, Schwartz's studies have recently shown that this is not the case [3-61].

SODIUM DEPLETION

Sodium depletion produces its renal effect largely on the basis of the associated depletion of extracellular volume. Decrease in glomerular filtration rate occurs with increased proximal tubular absorption of sodium. The lack of available sodium in the distal tubule impairs the kidney's ability to dilute the urine and to allow a normal water diuresis. Sodium depletion has also been found to inhibit excretion of bicarbonate [3-62]. Inability to conserve sodium may occur in various types of chronic renal disease [3-63], or after the release of obstructive uropathy [3-64].

HYPONATREMIA

The specific reaction of the kidney to a decrease in the serum sodium concentration is important in surgical patients. In such individuals hyponatremia is usually due to increased administration of water, with decreased water excretion due to postoperative elevation in ADH secretion, and not to decreased total body sodium stores. Thus the hyponatremic postoperative surgical patient will present a normal or elevated total body sodium but with a greatly increased total body water, so that the regulatory systems must handle an expanded volume and a lowered sodium concentration. Aldosterone secretion is inhibited by the expansion of the extracellular volume, and large amounts of sodium may be excreted in the urine even in the presence of hyponatremia. In addition, the excretion of free water is inhibited because of a decrease in the concentration of distal tubular sodium. It is thus possible for adequate urine output to be produced without altering the hypotonic state. Correction of this abnormality will occur in time by the withholding of electrolyte-free water [3-65]. Some improvement can be obtained by the administration of hypertonic saline or the withdrawal of water by peritoneal dialysis or intensive diuresis. During the diuresis isotonic salt solutions with adequate potassium should be infused [3-66]. The use of such a combination of sodium infusion and furosemide diuresis has produced good results in patients with cardiac failure and occasionally in patients with hepatic disease [3-67].

RENAL RESPONSE TO HEMORRHAGE

The response of the kidney to the stress of hemorrhage is of great importance to the surgeon. It has already been noted that a decrease in extracellular fluid volume causes increase in proximal tubular resorption of sodium, mediated presumably by hemodynamic and tissue-tension factors. There is also an increase in resorption of sodium mediated through the renin-angiotensin-aldosterone mechanism. Acute hypovolemia due to blood loss produces the same result even when the blood loss is of mild degree and the subject remains normotensive. Thus the loss of one 500 ml unit of blood by a normal individual will produce a decrease in urine volume and sodium excretion. Glomerular filtration rate will fall slightly, usually less than 10 per cent. With larger amounts of hemorrhage, still at normotensive levels, renal vasoconstriction occurs with a decrease in cortical blood flow and a more striking decrease in glomerular filtration rate [3-68, 3-69]. These changes are roughly parallel to changes in cardiac output [3-70]. With further blood loss, blood pressure falls and the effect of the decrease in perfusion pressure is added [3-71]. Under these conditions cortical blood flow is markedly reduced [3-72].

The stimuli for such changes in renal blood flow presumably arise within the pressure sensors of the cardiac chambers, aortic arch, carotid body, and perhaps within the kidney itself [3-55]. Both neural and humeral outflow appear to be important. Marked changes occur in the denervated or transplanted kidney [3-68, 3-73], although the sympathetic nervous system is required for the full response [3-74]. Prehemorrhage treatment of the kidney with vasodilators appears to ameliorate this response to some degree [3-75, 3-76]. Significant return of renal blood flow, glomerular filtration, and urinary excretion toward normal in the face of hypovolemia can be obtained by the use of the diuretics ethacrynic acid and furosemide [3-77]. Reinfusion of the blood lost apparently does not return renal blood-flow distribution to normal in dogs [3-78], whereas in humans renal blood flow and renal excretory function return promptly to normal. Intrarenal blood-flow distribution studies have not been done under these conditions in man [3-69].

RENAL RESPONSE TO SURGERY AND TRAUMA

Sodium Retention

Alterations in renal function due to major surgery or trauma have been noted for many years [3-78]. Water and sodium retention has been the usual finding in the first forty-eight hours following such injury. An increase in aldosterone secretion has been postulated as the cause for postoperative sodium retention. Studies have shown, however, that such retention may occur in the absence of the adrenal gland or under pretreatment with an aldosterone antagonist [3-43, 3-79]. Pre- and intraoperative expansion of the extracellular volume has produced an improvement in sodium excretion and correction of the deficit in free-water excretion [3-80, 3-81, 3-82].

Glomerular Filtration Rate (GFR)

In 1965 Dawson showed that glomerular filtration rate (GFR) decreased postoperatively in patients showing a clinically normal postoperative course [3-83]. This renal response to surgery has subsequently been confirmed [3-84]. In patients with a normal postoperative course and no oliguria, glomerular filtration rate falls an average of 30 per cent, returning to normal on the third to fourth postoperative day. This response to abdominal surgical trauma can be blocked by the intraoperative administration of ethacrynic acid. In such patients sodium and water retention is minimized.

Surgical trauma as well as accidental injury thus causes an alteration in renal function very similar to that caused by hypovolemia, and perhaps mediated in a similar manner. Preoperative dehydration, intraoperative hemorrhage, and the response to trauma are thus additive in their effects on the kidney, and each should be appropriately treated.

RENAL FAILURE

Renal failure is a condition in which the kidney cannot excrete the nitrogenous products of metabolism at a rate adequate to maintain normal serum levels. In addition to this glomerular failure, varying degrees of tubular damage or alteration may be present. The healthy human has a large reserve of kidney function, and the normal glomerular filtration rate of approximately 120 ml/min is four times the minimum required to maintain normal function.

Renal Reserve

Decrease in renal functional reserve can exist with normal blood urea nitrogen and creatinine levels, but with a decreased glomerular filtration rate. In a preoperative study of patients over 50 years of age, a considerable number were found with filtration rates below 50 ml/min [3-13]. In the absence of other renal disease it is assumed that arteriolar occlusion is the cause of this attrition of functioning nephron units. Since the normal response to major abdominal surgery and trauma involves a decrease of 30 per cent of GFR, it can be seen that a patient with a preoperative GFR of 40 to 50 ml/min may show a rising BUN (blood urea nitrogen) or serum creatinine for 3 to 4 days postoperatively, even though no permanent damage to the kidney has been produced. Patients with chronic renal disease of vascular or other type and who show preoperative elevation of BUN and creatinine have even lower filtration rates, usually below 30 ml/min. These patients are clearly at greater risk when operated upon.

Pathogenesis

Acute renal failure (acute tubular degeneration, shock kidney) is a term which has been used to indicate sudden decrease in renal function produced by prolonged hypotension, renal ischemia, damage from crushed tissue, injury due to transfusion reaction, and the like. The exact pathogenesis of such renal failure is still unclear, but the mechanisms of injury appear to be prolonged renal ischemia, obstruction of renal tubules by protein and cellular casts, and direct toxic effect on tubular cells from circulating foreign substances in blood or tubular fluid [3-84].

Oliguric and Nonoliguric Failure

Decrease in renal function may produce oliguria or anuria when the estimated filtration rate is below 5 to 6 ml/min, or may be associated with normal or even increased volumes of urine (nonoliguric renal failure, high-output failure). Nonoliguric renal failure presumably is associated with a slightly higher glomerular filtration rate—6 to 8 ml/min. In either case the level of glomerular filtration is insufficient to clear the blood of metabolic products, and the BUN and creatinine rise.

Oliguria appears to occur when some degree of tubular resorption occurs in the few functioning nephrons. Thus, at a GFR of 5 ml/min, the filtered volume would equal 7200 ml (5 × 1440 min per 24 hr). If proximal tubular resorption takes place, the final excreted urine volume may be only 150 to 200 ml per day. In some cases, however, a much higher percentage of filtrate is excreted, with the resulting increase in urine volume to normal or supranormal levels. In such patients with high-output failure, clearance of water and potassium is enhanced, although nitrogen clearance is not. These patients are more easily treated, since fluid and potassium excretion approach normal.

Renal Blood Flow

Renal blood-flow studies in these patients have shown a decrease of total renal blood flow with a particular decrease in cortical flow [3-85]. This decrease in cortical blood flow appears to occur whether renal failure is caused by ischemia [3-86] or by nephrotoxic substances [3-87].

Results of Inadequate Renal Function

The results of renal failure are the retention of metabolic products within the body and the inability to excrete water and electrolytes if oliguria or anuria exists. Widespread alteration in cellular metabolism occurs. This may be due to hydrogen-ion retention with decrease in intracellular pH [3-88]. Insulin action may be inhibited with alterations in glucose metabolism [3-89]. Membrane transport of sodium and potassium is affected. Alteration in amino acid metabolism may produce elevated levels of abnormal metabolites such as guanidinosuccinic acid [3-90]. This substance has been shown to produce many of the symptoms associated with uremia when injected into animals. Changes in capillary permeability appear to occur during acute renal failure [3-91], and wound healing is delayed in experimental animals [3-92]. These abnormalities can all be reversed by appropriate dialysis, or upon return of adequate renal function [3-93].

Complicating Effect of Body Tissue Injury

Renal failure can occur in any situation where renal perfusion is decreased, resulting in ischemia of renal tissue cells. A further result of decreased renal perfusion is enhancement of tubular resorption of sodium and water with increase in concentration of tubular fluid. When direct tissue damage with release of intracellular material is added, both the incidence and the severity of the renal failure increase. Cameron et al have reported an incidence of renal failure of 2.4 per cent in burn patients. In patients with greater than 15 per cent body surface burn, renal failure occurred in 16 per cent [3-94]. The incidence of renal failure is higher after injuries producing a great deal of tissue crushing, following tissue destruction due to sepsis, and after cardiopulmonary bypass [3-95].

PREVENTION OF RENAL FAILURE

Therapy at the onset of acute renal failure is directed toward producing a diuresis if possible.

Diuresis

INDICATIONS
Indications for therapy are the persistence of a urinary output of less than 20 ml/hr for more than two hours after adequate replacement

of any volume deficits. Agents used in the treatment of oliguria are mannitol and the diuretic agents, furosemide and ethacrynic acid.

MANNITOL

Mannitol is a six-carbon alcohol of molecular weight 182 which remains in the extracellular fluid. It is excreted almost completely unchanged in the urine. The diuretic effect of mannitol is apparently accomplished by the filtration of the molecule and its presence in the tubular fluid. Since mannitol cannot be resorbed from the tubule, an obligatory solute diuresis is produced. This diuresis produces a hyperosmolar urine of 400 to 600 milliosmoles per liter. In the doses usually employed in man, urine sodium concentrations are approximately one-half those of the plasma and replacement should be calculated accordingly.

Mannitol as usually given is a hypertonic solution. The initial reaction in the patient is an increase in intravascular water caused by the introduction of this solution. Plasma volume may be acutely expanded and central venous pressure may rise rapidly. Acute cardiac decompensation has been produced in this manner and should be guarded against. Mannitol is effective in the prevention and treatment of posttraumatic and postoperative renal failure [3-96, 3-97]. It is effective in the hydropenic states [3-98], but is less so in states of acute hypovolemia [3-77].

Mannitol can increase renal blood flow by decreasing renal vascular resistance in a manner yet not well understood. No increase in glomerular filtration rate occurs, and the diuresis produced is essentially a tubular phenomenon [3-99, 3-100]. There are no known permanent effects on the kidney, even from large doses, although vacuolization of tubular cells may appear [3-101]. Mannitol is a good osmotic diuretic which should be used initially in cases of oliguria and which can be expected to produce a diuresis in a high percentage of cases. Certain cases, however, are resistant to mannitol, presumably because the filtration rate is so low that adequate mannitol does not reach the tubule. Usually a test dose of 12.5 gm of mannitol intravenously will produce a diuresis if one is to be obtained. Further mannitol should not be given as the increase in circulating volume can be dangerous.

ETHACRYNIC ACID AND FUROSEMIDE

Ethacrynic acid [2,3-dichloro-4-(2-methylene butyl) phenoxyacetic acid] and fruosemide [4-chloro-N-(2-furylmethyl)5-sulfamylanthranilic acid] are two diuretics with great potency and very similar action. Both of these agents increase renal blood flow by decreasing renal vascular resistance [3-102, 3-103, 3-104]. They also produce an increase in filtration rate, an effect which occurs even in the hydropenic or hypovolemic state [3-77]. Sodium resorption is blocked in both proximal and distal renal tubules, and the excreted fraction of filtered sodium can rise as high as 30 per cent. Alteration of intrarenal blood flow distribution has been shown following administration of ethacrynic acid [3-105].

The urine produced during diuresis with ethacrynic acid or furosemide contains sodium in a concentration of 75 to 90 mEq/liter. Potassium is present in concentration of 8 to 10 mEq/liter. In a prolonged diuresis significant losses of magnesium and calcium are also encountered. Replacement of volume, if required, must be in accord with these losses. One-half normal saline with additional potassium chloride has been used, using magnesium and calcium supplements at intervals. The loss of calcium following such diuresis has been used as a treatment for acute hypercalcemic crisis. At present this is the most effective way to acutely reduce the serum calcium level short of parathyroidectomy.

Ethacrynic acid and furosemide have been shown to be capable of producing a diuresis after failure of mannitol. If usual doses of 40 to 50 mg do not initiate diuresis, larger doses may be tried. Successful diuresis has occurred after massive doses of furosemide [3-106, 3-107] or ethacrynic acid [3-94, 3-108, 3-109]. Occasional reports of cardiac irregularity following the use of ethacrynic acid have been documented and both ethacrynic acid and furosemide have caused transient deafness [3-110]. In general, however, these drugs are remarkably free of toxic side effects.

It is difficult to assess whether these diuretics actually shorten the recovery time of acute renal failure or simply convert oliguric to nonoliguric failure. Since recovery appears to be related to the washing out of tubular casts, and since these diuretics do increase tubular flow, it is logical to use them early in the course of renal failure as prophylaxis or therapy.

ESTABLISHED RENAL FAILURE

Mortality

The mortality of acute renal failure varies dramatically depending upon the etiologic circumstances. Derot et al, in a series of 647 cases treated from 1962 to 1964, showed a mortality of 0 to 7 per cent when renal failure was associated with transfusion reaction, abortion, drug toxicity, or mechanical obstruction. The mortality from renal failure associated with shock, surgery, and trauma, however, ranged from 60 to 87 per cent. These authors, in addition, confirmed the high mortality of renal failure associated with hepatic insufficiency, 59 per cent in their series [3-111].

Recovery Pattern

Recovery from acute renal failure will usually occur with time. The glomerular filtration rate gradually increases until metabolites can be adequately cleared from the plasma. Tubular function may remain abnormal for long periods of time. As long as one year later the response to injected vasopressin may be abnormal. The adequacy of recovery from acute renal failure is related to the level of renal function which existed prior to the insult. A return to approximately 80 per cent of the prefailure filtration rate can be expected.

Therapy

GENERAL SUPPORT

The management of the patient in renal failure requires careful fluid balance, recording of daily weights, and an understanding of the natural history of the syndrome. Measurement of creatinine clearance should be done frequently throughout the course. Treatment of the underlying condition must, of course, be given, and antibiotics administered, keeping in mind that renal excretion of such antibiotics is blocked, and therefore dosage must be adjusted accordingly. Intake should be limited to maintain serum electrolyte levels within the normal range. Blood-volume deficits should be made up with washed red cells. Protein metabolism should be minimized as much as possible by the administration of high carbohydrate intake orally or by central vein.

The blood levels of urea nitrogen, creatinine, and all electrolytes, especially potassium, must be monitored at suitable intervals. If the creatinine clearance is below 5, blood urea nitrogen will rise at approximately 30 mg per cent per 24 hr, and potassium will rise at approximately 1 mEq/liter/24 hr. If large energy demands are made upon the patient and large amounts of protein are being catabolized, these levels will rise much more rapidly. Acute changes in the serum potassium may take place if sudden alterations occur in cardiac output, circulating volume, and tissue perfusion. If tissue damage has taken place or if cell anoxia occurs due to hypoperfusion, potassium may rise precipitously.

Potassium levels of 5.0 mEq/liter or more should be considered dangerous and careful monitoring with frequent sampling of the blood level should be done. Cation exchange resins may be used by mouth, nasogastric tube, or by rectum to withdraw potassium, but the capacity and speed of this method is limited. Infusion of glucose-insulin solution may reduce serum potassium levels acutely, but the effect in temporary. Administration of calcium gluconate to maintain normal serum calcium levels may counter the cardiac effect of elevated potassium levels for a time. Unless renal excretion can be improved, however, continued rise in serum potassium is an indication for dialysis.

INDICATIONS FOR DIALYSIS

The decision to use dialysis must rest on several factors. First, if creatinine clearance is below 5 and remains at an extremely low level for one to two days, recovery can be expected to be prolonged and dialysis should be undertaken as a prophylactic measure. Repeated hemodialysis is most often needed. It must be stressed that the time for dialysis should be decided upon based on the rate of rise of urea nitrogen and potassium levels and on the underlying problems existing in the patient. If hemodialysis is unavailable or is considered to be contraindicated, peritoneal dialysis may be begun and can be effective for a period of three to five days. Experience has shown, however, that continuous peritoneal dialysis is required to maintain adequate clearance levels in the postsurgery and posttrauma patient. The contraindications to hemodialysis have become fewer and fewer, and this modality should be used in most cases.

SPECIAL PROBLEMS OF TISSUE DAMAGE

It should be emphasized that the septic, postsurgical, or posttrauma patient has a more acute problem when renal failure occurs than has the patient in whom renal failure is the only serious lesion. The high mortality reflects the serious nature of renal failure in the presence of tissue damage or sepsis. Dialysis must be performed early and frequently if survival is to be obtained [3-112, 3-113, 3-114].

METHODS OF MEASURING RENAL FUNCTION

Information concerning renal function can be obtained by relatively simple tests. The urinalysis with measurement of urinary protein and analysis of urinary sediment will give clues to chronic renal disease or infection. The ability to concentrate and dilute the urine is a measure of tubular function and can be measured by a postdehydration specimen or after administration of vasopressin. Normally the specific gravity will rise to 1.026 or over. Fixed low specific gravity after 6 to 8 hr of dehydration is an abnormal finding and indicates further diagnostic workup. Serum creatinine and urea nitrogen indicate the ability of the filtration mechanism to clear the serum of nitrogenous products of metabolism. It must be emphasized that normal levels of creatinine and urea indicate only that creatinine clearance is 30 ml/min or above. Such normal serum levels do not indicate actual renal reserve. A creatinine clearance, utilizing serum and urinary creatinine levels and a measured urinary volume is a more direct measurement of the level of glomerular filtration. Comparison of the urine to plasma creatinine concentration or urine to plasma urea concentration is a rough estimate of urinary concentrating power and thus of adequacy of tubular cell function. Values for U/P creatinine should be above 2.5 and for U/P urea should be above 10. Ratios below these levels indicate tubular cell damage.

PREOPERATIVE EVALUATION

Renal function should be assessed in any patient who is to undergo a major abdominal or general surgical procedure. A careful history should be obtained with special attention to previous renal disease or infection. Basic preoperative studies include the serum urea nitrogen, serum creatinine, and complete urinalysis. In a patient over age 50 or in a patient who is to undergo an operative procedure which may entail significant blood loss, or one who may suffer hypotensive episodes or need transfusion, or where extensive dissection and tissue damage may occur, preoperative creatinine clearance measurements should be done. This is most easily done on a 24-hr specimen, but can be performed on a specimen of any known time interval. Creatinine clearance measurements of less than 50 ml/min indicate the need for prophylactic diuresis during operation.

INTRAOPERATIVE CARE

Maintenance of normal ventilation and perfusion during an operative procedure will protect kidney function as well as the function of other organ systems. Blood-gas studies should be drawn at intervals to assure maintenance of normal ventilation. Volume replacement must be carefully given to maintain circulatory adequacy. Vasoconstricting pharmacologic agents including cyclopropane anesthesia, should be used only with knowledge of possible adverse renal effects. Function of the kidneys should be monitored during major procedures by measurement of urine output using an indwelling catheter.

Fluid Support

An acceptable routine of fluid support for major abdominal operations is that of the administration of 2 to 3 mEq of sodium per kilogram per hour. This amounts to 250 to 300 ml of Ringer's lactate solution per hour of operation in the normal adult. The appropriateness of this regimen should be checked by half hourly monitoring of urinary output.

Intraoperative Diuresis

A fall in urine output below 10 to 15 ml per half-hour in the absence of hypovolemia will indicate the need for diuresis. The administration of 12.5 gm of mannitol in 200 ml of Ringer's lactate solution should be tried. This diuretic will produce satisfactory renal blood flow and urinary excretion in most cases. Failure of response to this dose of mannitol indicates that ethacrynic acid or furosemide in doses of 50 or 40 mg, respectively, should be given. The drug can be added to 500 ml of glucose in water and infused at a rate of 100 ml/hr.

Prophylactic Diuresis

In patients with preoperative creatinine clearance levels below 50 ml/min, furosemide or ethacrynic acid diuresis should be started at the beginning of the operative procedure. Urine volumes produced by these diuretic agents must be replaced, volume for volume, with 0.45 per cent saline in order to prevent extracellular fluid dehydration.

POSTOPERATIVE CARE

Maintenance of the normal ventilation and perfusion state is equally important in the postoperative period if renal function is to be preserved. Patients with low preoperative clearance measurements should have interval-clearance measurements performed in the postoperative period. In any patient after serious surgery or trauma, especially involving hypovolemia, tissue damage, and/or transfusion, a decrease in renal function may occur. This may not always present with oliguria and in many cases urine output may remain normal. However, clearance levels may be low and serum creatinine and potassium may begin to rise. A high index of suspicion in such cases is the only protection. Urine to plasma creatinine or urea ratios may be used as a quick method of evaluating normality of renal function. Creatinine-clearance measurements give more precise information. Serum levels of urea nitrogen and potassium must be measured at frequent intervals.

Treatment of Postoperative Oliguria

Oliguria, defined as a urine volume of less than 20 ml/hr for two successive hours, should be treated vigorously. Assessment of the adequacy of circulating intravascular volume and of extracellular fluid volume must be made using all clinical indices; skin moisture, skin turgor, eyeball tension, and central venous pressure. Blood-volume measurements using isotopic methods are of value under these circumstances. If intravascular and extracellular volumes have been restored to normal and oliguria persists, diuresis with mannitol should be undertaken using a dose of 12.5 gm. If this dose does not produce an increase in urine volume, furosemide or ethacrynic acid should be used beginning with a dose of 40 mg for furosemide and 50 mg for ethacrynic acid. Using either of these agents, the dose may be doubled at successive one to two hours intervals until 600 mg or diuresis is reached. If renal failure becomes established, careful medical therapy with continuous monitoring of creatinine clearance, weight, and electrolyte and fluid balance must be undertaken. Dialysis is indicated as previously described if it appears that renal failure will be prolonged more than five to seven days.

REFERENCES

3-1.   Martino, J. A., and Earley, L. E.: Demonstration that renal hemodynamics and plasma oncotic pressure are mediators of the natriuretic response to volume expansion. J. Clin. Invest. 46:1092, 1967.

3-2. Barger, A. C., and Herd, J. A.: The renal circulation. New Engl. J. Med. 284:482, 1971.

3-3. Thorburn, G. D., Kopald, H. H., Herd, J. A., Hollenberg, M., O'Morchoe, C. C. C., and Barger, A. C.: Intrarenal distribution of nutrient blood flow determined with Krypton[85] in the unanesthetized dog. Circ. Res. 13:290, 1963.

3-4. Steiner, S. H., and King, R. D.: Nutrient renal blood flow and its distribution in the unanesthetized dog. J. Surg. Res. 10:133, 1970.

3-5. Sapirstein, L. A.: Regional blood flow by fractional distribution of indicators. Am. J. Physiol. 193:161, 1958.

3-6. Swann, H. G., and Prine, J. M.: Relation of intrarenal pressure to blood pressure and to perinephritic hypertension. Fed. Proc. 10: 134, 1951.

3-7. Swann, H. G., Hink, B. W., Koester, H., Moore, V., and Prine, J. M.: The intrarenal venous pressure. Science, 115:64, 1952.

3-8. McKenna, O. C., and Angelakos, E. T.: Adrenergic innervation of the canine kidney. Circ. Res. 22:345, 1968.

3-9. Ljungqvist, A., and Wagermark, J.: The adrenergic innervation of intrarenal glomerular and extra-glomerular circulatory routes. Nephron 7:218, 1970.

3-10. Tobias, G. J., McLaughlin, R. F., Jr., and Hopper, J., Jr.: Endogenous creatinine clearance. New Engl. J. Med. 266:317, 1962.

3-11. Philbin, P. E.: Correlation between short- and long-term endogenous creatinine clearance. Presented at annual meeting of the Am. Soc. of Nephrology, 1968 (program p. 50).

3-12. Goldring, W.: Clinical application of current tests of renal function. JAMA 153:1245, 1953.

3-13. Stahl, W. M., and Stone, A. M.: Prophylactic diuresis with ethacrynic acid for prevention of postoperative renal failure. Ann. Surg. 172:361, 1970.

3-14. Davidson, A. J., Talner, L. B., and Downs, W. M.: A study of the angiographic appearance of the kidney in an aging normotensive population. IVth International Congress of Nephrology, Stockholm, Sweden, 1969.

3-15. Goldsmith, R. S., Hyperparathyroidism. New Engl. J. Med. 281:367, 1969.

3-16. Thompson, D. D.: Renal excretion of calcium and phosphorus. Arch. Intern. Med. 103:832, 1959.

3-17. Heller, B. I., Hammarsten, J. F., and Stutzman, F. L.: Concerning the effects of magnesium sulfate on renal function, electrolyte excretion, and clearance of magnesium. J. Clin. Invest. 32:858, 1953.

3-18. Haitt, H. H., and Thompson, D. D.: The effects of parathyroid extract on renal function in man. J. Clin. Invest. 36:557, 1957.

3-19. Rector, F. C., Van Giesen, G., Kiil, F., and Seldin, D. W.: Influence of expansion of extracellular volume on tubular reabsorption of sodium independent of changes in glomerular filtration rate and aldosterone activity. J. Clin. Invest. 43:341, 1964.

3-20. Levinsky, N. G.: Nonaldosterone influences on renal sodium transport. Ann. N.Y. Acad. Sci. 139:295, 1966.

3-21. Wright, F. S., Brenner, B. M., Bennett, C. M., Keimowitz, R. I., Berliner, R. W., Schrier, R. W., Verroust, P. J., de Wardener, H. E., and Holzgreve, H.: Failure to demonstrate a hormonal inhibitor of proximal sodium resorption. J. Clin. Invest. 48:1107, 1969.

3-22. Earley, L. E., and Friedler, R. M.: Studies on the mechanism of natriuresis accompanying increased renal blood flow and its role in the renal response to extracellular volume expansion. J. Clin. Invest. 44:1857, 1965.

3-23. Earley, L. E., and Friedler, R. M.: The effects of combined renal vasodilatation and pressor agents on renal hemodynamics and the tubular reabsorption of sodium. J. Clin. Invest. 45:542, 1966.

3-24. Koch, K. M., Aynedijian, H. S., and Bank, N.: Effect of acute hypertension on sodium reabsorption by the proximal tubule. J. Clin. Invest. 47:1696, 1968.

3-25. Stahl, W. M.: Local and systemic factors affecting renal tissue tension. J. Surg. Res. 5:508, 1965.

3-26. Wada, T., Ogawa, M., Ishikawa, J., Yamauchi, M., Kato, E., and Asano, S.: The role of physical and humoral factors in saline diuresis: I. Influence of intrarenal interstitial fluid volume on proximal reabsorption. IVth International Congress of Nephrology, Stockholm, Sweden, 1969.

3-27. DeBono, E., and Mills, I. H.: Intrarenal monitoring of cardiac output in the regulation of sodium excretion. Lancet 2:1027, 1965.

3-28. Martino, J. A., and Earley, L. E.: Demonstration of a role of physical factors as determinants of the natriuretic response to volume expansion. J. Clin. Invest. 46:1963, 1967.

3-29. Gill, J. R., Jr., Mason, D. T., and Bartter, F. C.: Adrenergic nervous system in sodium metabolism: Effects of guanethidine and sodium-retaining steroids in normal man. J. Clin. Invest. 43:177, 1964.

3-30. Gill, J. R., and Bartter, F. C.: Adrenergic nervous system in sodium metabolism. II. Effects of guanethidine on the renal response to sodium deprivation in normal man. New Engl. J. Med. 275:1466, 1966.

3-31. Brenner, B. M., Falchuk, K. H., Keimowitz, R. I., and Berliner,

R. W.: The relationship between peritubular capillary protein concentration and fluid reabsorption by the renal proximal tubule. J. Clin. Invest. 48:1519, 1969.

3-32. Earley, L. E., Martino, J. A., and Friedler, R. M.: Factors affecting sodium reabsorption by the proximal tubule as determined during blockade of distal sodium reabsorption. J. Clin. Invest. 45:1668, 1966.

3-33. Schrier, R. W., and Earley, L. E.: Effects of hematocrit on renal hemodynamics and sodium excretion in hydropenic and volume-expanded dogs. J. Clin. Invest. 49:1656, 1970.

3-34. Suki, W. N., Yium, J. J., von Minden, M., Saller-Hebert, C., Eknoyan, G., and Martinez-Maldonado, M.: Acute treatment of hypercalcemia with furosemide. New Engl. J. Med. 283:836, 1970.

3-35. Eknoyan, G., Suki, W. N., Rector, F. C., Jr., and Seldin, D. W.: Functional characteristics of the diluting segment of the dog nephron and the effect of extracellular volume expansion on its resorptive capacity. J. Clin. Invest. 46:1178, 1967.

3-36. Weinstein, E., Manitus, A., and Epstein, F. H.: The importance of aerobic metabolism in the renal concentrating process. J. Clin. Invest. 48:1855, 1969.

3-37. Verney, E. B.: The antidiuretic hormone and the factors which determine its release. Proc. Royal Soc. London, Series B, 135:25, 1947.

3-38. Eggleton, M. G.: The diuretic action of alcohol in man. J. Physiol. 101:172, 1942.

3-39. Gupta, P. D., Sinclair, R., and Henry, J. P.: Role of atrial afferents in the tachycardia and increased ADH levels of moderate hemorrhage. (Abst.) Fed. Proc. 25:2161, 1966.

3-40. Share, L., and Levy, M. N.: Carotid sinus pulse pressure, a determinant of plasma antidiuretic hormone concentration. Am. J. Physiol. 211:721, 1966.

3-41. Segar, W. E., and Moore, W. W.: The regulation of antidiuretic hormone release in man. I. Effects of change in position and ambient temperature on blood ADH levels. J. Clin. Invest. 47:2143, 1968.

3-42. Moran, W. H., Jr., Miltenberger, F. W., Shuayb, W. A., and Zimmerman, B.: The relationship of antidiuretic hormone secretion to surgical stress. Surgery 56:99, 1964.

3-43. Luttwak, E. M., and Saltz, N. J.: Studies on postoperative antidiuresis in adrenalectomized patients. Surg. Gynec. Obst. 115:312, 1962.

3-44. Dudley, H. F., Boling, E. A., LeQuesne, L. P., and Moore, F. D.: Studies on antidiuresis in surgery: Effects of anesthesia, surgery and posterior pituitary antidiuretic hormone on water metabolism in man. Ann. Surg. 140:354, 1954.

3-45. Lauson, H. D.: Antidiuretic hormone. Fed. Proc. 24:731, 1965.

3-46. Buckalew, V. M., Jr., Walker, B. R., Puschett, J. B., and Goldberg, M.: Effects of increased sodium delivery on distal tubular sodium resorption with and without volume expansion in man. J. Clin. Invest. 49:2336, 1970.

3-47. Sharp, G. W. G., and Leaf, A.: Mechanism of action of aldosterone. Physiol. Rev. 46:593, 1966.

3-48. Tobian, L.: Renin release and its role in renal function and the control of salt balance and arterial pressure. Fed. Proc. 26:48, 1967.

3-49. Grundy, H. M., Simpson, S. A., and Tait, J. F.: Isolation of a highly active mineralocorticoid from beef adrenal extract. Nature 169:795, 1952.

3-50. Davis, J. O., Carpenter, C. C. J., Ayers, C. R., Holman, J. E., and Bahn, R. C.: Evidence for secretion of an aldosterone stimulating hormone by the kidney. Fed. Proc. 20 (Suppl. 7):178, 1961.

3-51. Laragh, J. H., and Stoerk, H. C.: A study of the mechanism of secretion of the sodium-retaining hormone (aldosterone). J. Clin. Invest. 36:383, 1957.

3-52. Hartroft, P. M., and Edelman, R.: Renal juxtaglomerular cells in sodium deficiency; in J. H. Moyer and M. Fuchs (eds.): Edema —mechanisms and management. Philadelphia, Saunders, 1960, pp. 63–68.

3-53. Bartter, F. C., Liddle, G. W., Duncan, L. E., Jr., Barber, J. K., and Delea, C.: The regulation of aldosterone secretion in man: The role of fluid volume. J. Clin. Invest. 35:1306, 1956.

3-54. Ajzen, H., Simmons, J. L., and Woods, J. W.: Renal vein renin and juxtaglomerular activity in sodium-depleted subjects. Circ. Res. 17:130, 1965.

3-55. Stahl, W. M.: The pressure control of renin release by the kidney. Vasc. Dis. 3:180, 1966.

3-56. Cooke, C. R., Brown, T. C., Zacherle, B. J., and Walker, W. G.: The effect of altered sodium concentration in the distal nephron segments on renin release. J. Clin. Invest. 49:1630, 1970.

3-57. Tobian, L., Braden, M., and Maney, J.: The effect of unilateral renal denervation on the secretion of renin. Fed. Proc. 49:405. 1965.

3-58. Steinmetz, P. R.: Excretion by acid by the kidney—functional organization and cellular aspects of acidification. New Engl. J. Med. 278:1102, 1968.

3-59. Berliner, R. W.: Ion exchange mechanisms in the nephron. Circulation 21:892, 1960.

3-60. Lotspeich, W. D.: Metabolic aspects of acid-base change. Science 155:1066, 1967.

3-61. Schwartz, W. B., and Relman, A. S.: Effects of electrolyte disorders on renal structure and function. New Engl. J. Med. 276:383, 1967.

3-62. Schwartz, W. B., van Ypersele de Strihou, C., and Kassirer, J. P.: Role of anions in metabolic alkalosis and potassium deficiency. New Engl. J. Med. 279:630, 1968.

3-63. Coleman, A. J., Arias, M., Carter, N. W., Rector, F. C., Jr., and Seldin, D. W.: The mechanism of salt wastage in chronic renal disease. J. Clin. Invest. 45:1116, 1966.

3-64. Muldowney, F. P., Duffy, G. J., Kelly, D. G., Duff, F. A., Harrington, C., and Freaney, R.: Sodium diuresis after relief of obstructive uropathy. New Engl. J. Med. 274:1294, 1966.

3-65. Leaf, A., Bartter, F. C., Santos, R. F., and Wrong, O.: Evidence in man that urinary electrolyte loss induced by pitressin is a function of water retention. J. Clin. Invest. 32:868, 1953.

3-66. Leaf, A.: The clinical and physiologic significance of the serum sodium concentration. New Engl. J. Med. 267:24, 1962.

3-67. Cohen, I.: The effect of sodium loading on diuresis in patients with low serum sodium due to water overload. IVth International Congress of Nephrology, Stockholm, Sweden, 1969, p. 208.

3-68. Berne, R. M., and Levy, M. N.: Effects of acute reduction in cardiac output on the denervated kidney. Am. J. Physiol. 171:558, 1952.

3-69. Stone, A. M., and Stahl, W. M.: Renal effects of hemorrhage in normal man. Ann. Surg. 172:825, 1970.

3-70. Stahl, W. M.: The relationship of renal excretion of sodium and water to atrial pressures and cardiac output. J. Clin. Invest. 44:1100, 1965.

3-71. Stahl, W. M.: Renal regulation of solute and water excretion: The role of hemodynamic changes. Invest. Urol. 3:130, 1965.

3-72. Carrière, S., Thorburn, G. D., O'Morchoe, C. C. C., and Barger, C.: Intrarenal distribution of blood flow in dogs during hemorrhagic hypotension. Circ. Res. 19:167, 1966.

3-73. Rosen, S. M., Truniger, B., Kriek, H. R., Oken, D. E., Murray, J. E., and Merrill, J. P.: Intrarenal distribution of blood flow in normal and autotransplanted dog kidneys. Effect of hemorrhagic hypotension and mannitol. J. Clin. Invest. 44:1092, 1965.

3-74. Gill, J. R., Jr., and Casper, A. G. T.: Role of the sympathetic nervous system in the renal response to hemorrhage. J. Clin. Invest. 48:915, 1969.

3-75. Gump, F. E., Magill, T., Thal, A. P., and Kinney, J. M.: Regional adrenergic blockade by intra-arterial injection of phenoxybenzamine. Surg. Gynec. Obst. 127:319, 1968.

3-76. Carrière, S., and Daigneault, B.: Effect of retransfusion after hemorrhagic hypotension on intrarenal distribution of blood flow in dogs. J. Clin. Invest. 49:2205, 1970.

3-77. Stone, A. M., and Stahl, W. M.: Effect of ethacrynic acid and furosemide on renal function in hypovolemia. Ann. Surg. 174:1, 1971.

3-78. Moore, F. D., and Ball, M. R.: The metabolic response to surgery. Am. Lecture Ser. Publ. 132. Springfield, Ill., Thomas, 1952.

3-79. Kay, R. G.: The effect of an aldosterone antagonist upon the electrolyte response to surgical trauma. Brit. J. Surg. 55:266, 1968.

3-80. Gann, D. S., and Wright, H. K.: Augmentation of sodium excretion in postoperative patients by expansion of the extracellular fluid volume. Surg. Gynec. Obst. 118:1024, 1964.

3-81. Schlegel, J. U., Anderson, F. W., Madsen, P. O., and Betheil, J. J.: The altered response to sodium loading in several severely burned individuals after initial treatment with hypertonic sodium containing fluids. Surg. Gynec. Obst. 99:187, 1954.

3-82. Wright, H. K., and Gann, D. S.: Correction of defect in free water excretion in postoperative patients by extracellular fluid volume expansion. Ann. Surg. 158:70, 1963.

3-83. Dawson, J. L.: Post-operative renal function in obstructive jaundice: Effect of a mannitol diuresis. Brit. Med. J. 1:82, 1965.

3-84. Myers, J. K., Storrs, D., Miller, T. B., and Mueller, C. B.: The role of renal tubular flow in the pathogenesis of traumatic renal failure. Surg. Gynec. Obst. 123:1243, 1966.

3-85. Ladefoged, J., and Winkler, K.: Hemodynamics in acute renal failure. Scand. J. Clin. Lab. Invest. 26:83, 1970.

3-86. Hollenberg, N. K., Epstein, M., Rosen, S. M., Basch, R. I., Oken, D. E., and Merrill, J. P.: Acute oliguric renal failure in man: evidence for preferential renal cortical ischemia. Medicine, 47: 455, 1968.

3-87. Hollenberg, N. K., Adams, D. F., Oken, D. E., Abrams, H. L., and Merrill, J. P.: Acute renal failure due to nephrotoxins. Renal hemodynamic and angiographic studies in man. New Engl. J. Med. 282:1329, 1970.

3-88. Halperin, M. L., Connors, H. P., Relman, A. S., and Karnovsky, M. L.: Factors that control the effect of pH on glycolysis in leukocytes. J. Biol. Chem. 244:384, 1969.

3-89. Walker, B. G., Phear, D. N., Martin, F. I. R., and Baird, C. W.: Inhibition of insulin by acidosis. Lancet 2:964, 1963.

3-90. Cohen, B. D.: Guanidine retention and the urea cycle. IVth International Congress of Nephrology, Stockholm, Sweden, 1969.

3-91. Gibson, D. G.: Haemodynamic factors in the development of acute pulmonary oedema in renal failure. Lancet 2:1217, 1966.

3-92. Nayman, J.: Effect of renal failure on wound healing in dogs. Response to hemodialysis following uremia induced by uranium nitrate. Ann. Surg. 164:227, 1966.

3-93.   Merrill, J. P., and Hampers, C. L.: Uremia (in two parts). New
         Engl. J. Med. 282:953, and 282:1014, 1970.

3-94.   Cameron, J. S., Miller-Jones, C. M. H., and Trounce, J. R.: Renal
         function and renal failure in severely burnt patients. Proc.
         Europ. Dialysis and Transplant Assoc. 2:27, 1965.

3-95.   Kulatilake, A. E., and Shackman, R.: Acute renal failure in cardio-
         vascular surgery. Proc. Europ. Dialysis and Transplant Assoc.
         2:35, 1965.

3-96.   Boba, A., Landmesser, C. M., and Powers, S. R., Jr.: Prophylactic
         aspects of posttraumatic and postoperative renal failure. New
         York J. Med. 63:812, 1963.

3-97.   Barry, K. G.: Post-traumatic renal shutdown in humans: Its pre-
         vention and treatment by the intravenous infusion of mannitol.
         Mil. Med. 128:224, 1963.

3-98.   Berger, B., Evers, W., and Mueller, C. B.: Mannitol-induced
         diuresis in hydropenic men. Surgery 64:381, 1968.

3-99.   Stahl, W. M.: Effect of mannitol on the kidney. Changes in intra-
         renal hemodynamics. New Engl. J. Med. 272:381, 1965.

3-100.   Murphy, G. P., and Gagnon, J. A.: The alterations in glomerular
         filtration rate, osmolar, and free water clearance during mannitol
         osmotic diuresis. J. Urol. 92:17, 1964.

3-101.   Stuart, F. P., Torres, E., Fletcher, R., Crocker, D., and Moore,
         F. D.: Effects of single, repeated and massive mannitol infusion
         in the dog: Structural and functional changes in kidney and
         brain. Ann. Surg. 172:190, 1970.

3-102.   Hook, J. B., Blatt, A. H., Brody, M. J., and Williamson, H. E.:
         Effects of several saluretic-diuretic agents on renal hemodynamics.
         J. Pharm. Exper. Ther. 154:667, 1966.

3-103.   Eng, K., and Stahl, W. M.: Correction of the renal hemodynamic
         changes produced by surgical trauma. Ann. Surg. 174:19, 1971.

3-104.   Ludens, J. H., Hook, J. B., Brody, M. J., and Williamson, H. E.:
         Enhancement of renal blood flow by furosemide. J. Pharm.
         Exper. Ther. 16:456, 1968.

3-105.   Epstein, M., Hollenberg, N. K., Buttmann, R. I., and Merrill, J. P.:
         The effect of ethacrynic acid and chlorothiazide on the intrarenal
         distribution of blood flow (IDBF) in man. Am. Soc. Nephrology,
         IIIrd Annual Meeting, Washington, D.C., 1969.

3-106.   Sullivan, J. F., Kreisberger, C., and Mittal, A.: Effect of massive
         intravenous furosemide doses in acute oliguria. Am. Soc.
         Nephrology, IIIrd Annual Meeting, Washington, D.C., 1969.

3-107.   Shalhoub, R. J., Velasquez, M. T., and Antoniou, L. D.: Reversal
         of surgical oliguric states by furosemide or ethacrynic acid. Am.
         Soc. Nephrology, IIIrd Annual Meeting, Washington, D.C.,
         1969.

3-108.   Swartz, C., Chinitz, J., Onesti, G., Kim, K., Ramirez, O., and

Brest, A. N.: Ethacrynic acid in acute renal failure. Am. Soc. Nephrology, Third Annual Meeting, Washington, D.C., 1969.

3-109. Kjellstrand, C. M.: Ethacrynic acid in acute renal failure. Am. Soc. Nephrology, Third Annual Meeting, Washington, D.C., 1969.

3-110. Schwartz, G. H., David, D. S., Riggio, R. R., Stenzel, K. H., and Rubin, A. L.: Ototoxicity induced by furosemide. New Engl. J. Med. 282:1413, 1970.

3-111. Derot, M., Legrain, M., and Jacobs, C.: Indications respectives du rein artificiel et da la dialyse peritoneale dans le traitement de l'insuffisance renale aiguë (a propos de 537 observations). Proc. Europ. Dialysis and Transplant Assoc. 2:44, 1965.

3-112. Burns, R. O., Henderson, L. W., Hager, E. B., and Merrill, J. P.: Peritoneal dialysis. Clinical experience. New Engl. J. Med. 267: 1060, 1962.

3-113. Lamprecht, C., and Kessel, M.: Peritoneal dialysis in the treatment of burns. IVth International Congress of Nephrology, Stockholm, Sweden, 1969.

3-114. Aye, M. M., Kulatilake, A. K., and Shackman, R.: Peritoneal dialysis in surgery. Proc. Europ. Dialysis and Transplant Assoc. 2:49, 1965.

4

SKIN

PRIMARY FUNCTION

The most obvious interface between man and his surroundings is the outer covering of the body—the skin. This layer has developed as an organ for protection of man and animal from the environment. Specialized functions within the skin enable this organ to buffer extreme physical and chemical changes in the environment and make it possible for the homeothermic animal to maintain a relatively steady internal state. In man, the skin is distinguished from other animals in that it has no layer of insulating fur and that it is equipped with thermal-sensitive sweat glands. In the average adult the skin weighs approximately 3 kg and has a surface area of nearly two square meters.

ANATOMY

The skin is composed of two distinct tissue layers, the epidermis and the dermis. The epidermis develops during fetal existence from the ectoderm while the dermis is developing from the mesoderm. In spite of development from different layers, these two dermal cell types become interdependent in the mature organism. The skin is attached to the underlying musculoskeletal structures by fibrous tissue bands. These traverse the subcutaneous tissues where variable amounts of fat accumulate.

EPIDERMIS

The epidermis is a stratified epithelium which forms a uniform layer over most of the body surfaces. This layer measures from 0.06 to 0.1 mm in thickness, except on the palms and soles where the stratum corneum or keratinized surface layer is greatly thickened. Ninety to ninety-five per cent of the epidermal cells are keratinocytes, cells which differentiate toward the surface to produce the stratum corneum. The remaining epidermal cells are melanocytes which are involved in the production of skin pigment.

The entire process of differentiation of epidermal keratinocytes from basal layer to stratum corneum cells requires 28 days to complete. Thus the turnover time of skin epidermal cells is from six to seven times as long as that of intestinal epithelial cells. As the cell moves from the basal layer to the stratum corneum it becomes thin and flat, extending its surface area.

Each stratum corneum cell covers an area occupied by approximately 25 basal cells. The nucleus and cytoplasmic organelles disappear during this process, and the cell membrane increases in thickness to about 200 Å. In addition, the cell contains one or more fibrous proteins collectively called keratin. These lie in a system of filaments embedded in a continuous matrix and in a thickened cell membrane. Keratin appears to arise from two sources, from filaments already present in the differentiating cell, and from keratohyaline-containing granules found in the differentiating cells [4-1, 4-2].

Function of Epidermal Cells

The mature keratinocytes which comprise the stratum corneum possess unique biological characteristics, namely, thick cell membrane, absence of nucleus or any cell organelle, low water content, and high content of keratin. These special characteristics give this layer its particular protective characteristics: (1) low permeability to water and electrolytes, (2) high electrical impedance, (3) resistance to chemical injury due to keratin content, and (4) inhibition of bacterial proliferation due to the dry external surface.

Fluid Content of Stratum Corneum

The stratum corneum normally contains approximately 10 per cent water when the air has a relative humidity of 60 per cent. When water content is below 10 per cent, the skin looks excessively dry. As the relative humidity of the surroundings increases to 100 per cent, the water content of the stratum corneum increases to 70 to 80 per cent. The gross thickness of this layer changes also, from a normal of 15 microns at 60 per cent humidity to 48 microns at 100 per cent humidity [4-3, 4-4]. Under normal circumstances body water is continually passing through the stratum corneum, since the underlying subcutaneous tissues contain a higher percentage of water than the external layer. The 24-hr insensible loss by this route approximates 500 ml of water and maintains normal hydration (10 per cent) of the stratum corneum. With this degree of hydration the external layer maintains its normal supple quality.

Water and Electrolyte Transport

A vital function of this layer is its resistance to the passage of water and electrolytes. The permeability constant of the stratum corneum in cm/sec is 1.1×10^{-7} contrasted with the permeability constant of the erythrocyte membrane of 1.2×10^{-2}. The water flux through the membrane therefore is 1/100,000 of the water flux across the red cell membrane. The two membranes are very similar in their chemical composition, and their diffusion constants are much the same. The difference in permeability is therefore due to differences in thickness of the membrane, the stratum corneum normally measuring 15 microns while the red cell membrane measures 0.008 micron.

Molecular substances may be transported through the skin by three possible mechanisms. First, through the pyelosebaceous and sweat glands; second, through the intercellular space of the stratum corneum; third, directly through the keratinocytes of the stratum corneum. The pyelosebaceous follicles and sweat glands are invaginations of the epidermis. These are lined by stratum corneum only in their most superficial areas. The total surface area of all the pyelosebaceous and sweat glands, however, is only 1/100 to 1/1000 of the surface area of the entire body. Thus, although higher local fluxes may occur, this route seems to be less important except in two particular instances—first the initial stage of transepidermal transport, and second the transport of molecular substances with very low permeability [4-5].

Some substances may be transported through the skin by means of the intercellular spaces. This may occur in the case of certain electrolytes, since these are insoluble in the membrane of the keratinocyte.

Most electrolyte transport, however, occurs via eccrine glands [4-6]. In addition, the total volume of the intercellular space within the stratum corneum is 0.01–0.1 per cent of the volume of the stratum corneum. It thus would appear that most molecules are transported through the multiple layers of keratinocytes.

Transport across the stratum corneum is enhanced by increased temperature of the skin, apparently due to the effect of higher temperature in causing greater molecular activity. Solute substances which are lipid-soluble are also transported more rapidly, presumably due to the high lipid content of the membrane of the keratinocyte. Increased hydration of the stratum corneum also raises its permeability to four to five times normal. One explanation of this increased transport is the separation of the molecules of keratin protein by less tightly bound water, allowing molecular movements through the interstices. The stratum corneum is the most important layer limiting water transport through the skin, since the dermis is approximately 1000 times more permeable.

DERMIS

The dermis comprises the principal mass of the skin organ. It is made up primarily of noncellular fibroelastic connective tissue which encloses the glands and other appendages of the skin, and in addition contains nerves and blood vessels. The ground substance of the dermis also contains collagen and elastic fibers. The dermis varies in thickness from 1 to 4 mm, being thickest over the back, intermediate in thickness over the abdomen and thighs, and thinnest over the face and hands. The interface between dermis and epidermis consists of papillary projections of both layers interdigitating with each other, the "rete pegs."

Collagen

The wet weight of the dermis is made up of fibrous protein, the largest amount of which is collagen [4-7]. This substance, in the form of tropocollagen macromolecules, is organized into collagen fibers which normally lie in the dermis in a randomized arrangement, allowing the skin to be deformed by very little strain up to the point when the collagen fibers have become aligned in one direction. From this point on a rapidly increasing strain is required to produce further deformation of the skin. Thus the arrangement and mechanical properties of the collagen fibers allow small deformations to occur easily but cause large deformations to be resisted strongly [4-8].

Elastin

Elastic fibers are present in far fewer numbers than collagen fibers but lend an important characteristic to the dermal layer. These fibers provide the restoring forces necessary to return the collagen network to its original position. Elastic fibers tend to degenerate with age, producing loosening and wrinkling of the skin in the older person [4-9].

Blood Supply

The dermis encloses a network of blood vessels supplying dermal and epidermal layers. These blood vessels are arranged in a deep and superficial network with interconnecting vessels. The superficial dermal network sends loops into the papillary projections of the dermis [4-10]. The skin lymphatic plexus tends to parallel the vascular arrangement [4-11].

Thermal Regulation

In addition to supplying nutrient circulation to dermal and epidermal cells, the dermal vasculature is a vital component of the thermal regulatory mechanism of the body and participates actively in the inflammatory response. Nutritional blood flow has been estimated at 0.8 ml/min/100 ml of skin, or a total of 40 to 60 ml/min for the entire skin organ. At normal ambient temperatures, however, actual blood flow to the skin is approximately 500 ml/min. Exposure to a warm thermal environment may increase skin blood flow as much as six to eight times, while exposure to a cold external environment reduces blood flow by an equal amount [4-12]. Total skin blood flow, therefore, may vary from approximately 300 ml/min to over 3000 ml/min, with accompanying changes in demand for cardiac output. Such changes in cutaneous circulation produce secondary alterations in renal function, with an increase in urine volume occurring due to cold exposure and a decrease in urine volume during exposure to a warm environment. Factors which increase heat production within the body cause a compensatory increase in skin circulation so that a constant internal temperature can be maintained [4-13].

Nerves

The dermal layer contains a variety of nerve fibers and endings which relate to the sensation of cold and hot and transmit information of pain or itching. Large mechanoreceptors (Meissner and Pacinian corpuscles) are present. Adrenergic nerves run to the erector pili muscles. Cholinergic fibers supply the eccrine sweat glands. Adrenergic and possibly cholinergic fibers supply smooth muscles in the blood vessel wall.

Sweat Glands

The normal adult has from two to three million eccrine sweat glands in his skin. These represent a highly developed mechanism for thermoregulation. The density of occurrence of the eccrine sweat glands varies from one region of the body to the other, ranging from 130/sq cm on the leg to 600/sq cm on the sole of the foot. Each gland consists of a secretory and a ductal element, well supplied with blood vessels and nerve endings.

PRODUCTION OF SWEAT

The eccrine sweat gland responds to cholinergic and adrenergic substances, with the production of a hypotonic solution. The total volume of sweat can reach 2–3 liters/hr for short periods of time. Function of the excretory and ductal elements of the sweat glands mimic, to a certain degree, glomerular and tubular function in the kidney. Active secretion of lactate and hydrogen ion occurs. Hydrogen ion is resorbed after reaction with bicarbonate in the presence of carbonic anhydrase. Sodium, potassium, and chloride are secreted during the passage of the solution down the ductal segment, where some resorption of sodium also occurs. The total amount of sodium lost depends somewhat on the rate of sweat production, as the resorptive capabilities of the transporting segment can be exceeded [4-14]. Resorption of sodium in the transporting segment is responsive to aldosterone, increased resorption resulting when aldosterone levels are elevated.

THERMAL REGULATION BY SWEATING

Stimulation of the production of sweat occurs when body core temperature rises. This apparently is mediated through temperature-sensitive centers in the hypothalamus. Altered function of the hypothalamic temperature sensors may be found in fever states where sweating is not induced at the usual core-temperature level. An immediate response with the production of sweat occurs following body exercise. In addition, the eccrine sweat glands of the palms and soles and those in the axillae respond to psychogenic stimuli.

COORDINATED THERMAL REGULATION BY THE SKIN

The skin participates in thermal regulation by controlling the radiant and convective transfer of heat with the environment. At ambient temperatures less than 37°C, heat is lost by both these means to the environment, whereas when the ambient temperature is above 37°C heat is gained. Body heat is also lost through the evaporation of sweat, at the rate of 2260 joules/gm of water evaporated.

When increased body heat production occurs, heat is transmitted via the blood stream to the skin. The cutaneous circulation may increase heat loss by increasing blood volume in the skin and by increasing blood flow. With vasodilatation, the circulating blood approaches the skin surface. Heat conduction through skin layers is thus eliminated as a limiting factor. However, when vasoconstriction in the skin occurs to conserve body heat, the distance between the cutaneous blood flow and the environment is increased and conduction may become a limiting factor [4-15].

INFLAMMATION

Alteration in the function of the skin as an organ of thermoregulation and protection may occur as a result of injury or because of cutaneous inflammation. In these situations a basic pattern of response occurs. Vasoconstriction occurs immediately, lasting approximately 5 to 10 min and is followed by arteriolar vasodilatation. This reaction apparently depends on local release of histamine, serotonin, and kinins, and perhaps upon exhaustion of local tissue epinephrine stores. Skin flow may increase tenfold due to such vasodilatation [4-16]. Leukocytes become sticky and adhere to the endothelium of small vessels, especially veins. Permeability of the venules is increased with transvenular leakage of plasma. Such leakage apparently occurs between endothelial cells as separation of these cells can be seen on electron microscopy [4-17]. Leukocytes move into the tissue spaces. Edema of the tissue may increase as lymph channels are plugged with fibrin. Local enzyme action increases with release of proteases from cells and collagenases from leukocytes.

The severity of the inflammatory response depends upon the severity of the initial injury, the degree of tissue damage, the presence of bacterial infection, and the ability of the circulation of the organism to bring adequate oxygen, nutriment, and white blood cells to the local area.

SYSTEMIC EFFECTS OF SKIN INJURY

The systemic effect of the skin injury depends in great part on the area of skin involved. Increase in cardiac output has been noted in patients with localized but large areas of inflammation or abscess [4-18]. More severe and more widespread skin damage due to thermal injury produces serious metabolic changes. Even superficial second-degree burns with loss of the epidermis and cutaneous vasodilatation of significant areas (greater than 15 per cent) of the body surface allow increased water permeability and increased evaporative heat loss [4-19]. Hyperdynamic demands are placed on the circulation by increased cutaneous blood flow.

Full-thickness skin injury of large areas of the body places a greater demand on the total organism. Elevation of cardiac index to two times normal may occur, apparently due to an increased blood flow through the damaged areas [4-20]. Heat loss due to evaporative water transfer from damaged skin areas may impose a large requirement on endogenous heat production. In severe burns this energy requirement may be 150 to 200 per cent of the normal resting energy expenditure [4-21], and may occur across a burn eschar [4-22], or across granulation tissue [4-23]. The healed burn scar may itself alter thermal regulation [4-24]. Caloric needs due to insensible loss may range up to 6000 calories/sq m/day [4-25]. Occlusion of the damaged skin by the application of a nonpermeable covering reduces the water loss and caloric demands. This, however, may be associated with significant hyperthermia, and introduces serious danger of infection as bacteria proliferate beneath the covering. Early closure of severe wounds, especially burns, by suture or skin grafting, restores the normal protective skin covering [4-26].

WOUND HEALING

Prompt and complete healing of the incised skin wound is desired following operation or injury. Repair of the incised wound takes place by the ingrowth of fibroblasts and capillaries during the first three to five days after wounding. Fibrin and clot are lysed and removed by the circulation. Fibrinolysis occurs due to plasminogin activator produced by the endothelial cells. At four to five days, ground substance appears and collagen synthesis begins.

Epithelial coverage occurs by mobilization of cells from the basal epidermal layers and their migration to the surface or across denuded areas. Mitosis of these cells occurs with increase in the number of available cells. Differentiation follows to produce keratin-containing keratinocytes and restore the stratum corneum [4-27, 4-28]. Such epithelial mobilization and migration occurs before connective tissue regeneration is initiated. With epithelialization, molding of the collagen repair of the wound occurs, presumably due to collagenases released from epithelial cells. Mitosis and migration occur until normal complete covering by epithelial cells is achieved. Cessation of such mitotic activity apparently occurs due to contact inhibition.

Wound strength develops due to proliferation of fibroblasts and the deposition of collagen. The formation of tropocollagen molecules and collagen fibrils occurs beginning with the fourth to sixth day. Wound strength continues to increase over the ensuing weeks due to intramolecular and intermolecular cross-linkage of collagen fibers and remodeling of these fibers to give a stronger network. The effect of the mucopolysacchrides of the ground substance on such remodeling of collagen is at present uncertain [4-29].

Interference with Healing

Interference with proper wound healing may occur due to interference with cell mitosis. Shock has been noted to inhibit epidermal mitosis, presumably due to increase in circulating levels of cortisone and epinephrine. Both of these substances are powerful mitotic inhibitors. Starvation also inhibits mitosis in epidermal cells, presumably due to an increase in circulating epinephrine. The combination of epinephrine and another factor termed a *chalone* is postulated to account for all of the mitotic response seen in the healing wound [4-27]. The tensile strength of wounds can be adversely affected by protein depletion, by prolonged hypovolemia, by generalized hypercoagulability, by vasoconstriction, and by other mechanisms including hormones and irradiation [4-30]. A common factor in these states may be the interference with adequate oxygen delivery to cells [4-31]. The presence of a normal bacterial flora apparently does not inhibit wound healing as measured by the contraction of an open wound [4-32]. Wounds in the germ-free animal do show less inflammatory response, however.

WOUND INFECTION

Interruption of the integrity of the skin due to trauma or surgical operation provides a mode of entry for infectious agents. Factors involved in the production of infections of surgical or traumatic wounds may be conveniently divided into three groups: elements of wound contamination, factors within the wound itself which predispose to infection, and the metabolic condition of the host. Traumatic wounds are frequently seriously contaminated at the time of injury. Prevention of contamination is desirable in the case of a surgical incision.

Skin Preparation for Incision

Preparation of the skin of both the patient and the surgeon has received a great deal of attention as a means for reducing possible contamination during surgery. Prior to the development of improved skin detergents and antiseptics, contamination from the skin of the patient or the surgeon was considered a serious problem [4-33]. It would appear, however, that the use of solutions containing organic iodide reduces the resident bacteria in the skin of patients and on the hands of surgeons to such low levels that this is no longer the most important consideration [4-34]. Skin contact of a povidone-iodine solution for one minute would appear to be adequate to reduce bacteria counts to extremely low levels, and if this solution remains on the skin during the operative procedure, continuous antibacterial action will occur. Likewise, a five-minute surgical scrub with similar material provides protection for at least two hours within the surgical rubber gloves.

Contamination

Following wound closure, direct contamination of the wound from without almost never occurs if wound edges are well vitalized, properly approximated, and exposed to their normal environment, the surrounding air. Contamination can occur if wounds cannot be closed immediately, as in the case of burns, or if foreign bodies such as drains, tubes, and the like traverse the intact skin. Percutaneous sutures may provide a mode of entry for bacteria [4-35, 4-36]. The high percentage of infections in indwelling plastic catheters is an indication of this problem [4-37, 4-38].

Cross Infection

When wounds cannot be closed physiologically, it is quite clear that contamination may be transmitted from one patient to another through the air or by equipment which is used by the patient. Equipment such as sinks, lavatories, floor and corridor cleaning equipment, vacuum cleaners, bed linen, bed pans, and respirators, have clearly been shown to harbor pathogenic bacteria [4-39, 4-40].

Endogenous Bacteria

Colonization by endogenous bacteria does occur and may be significant under certain conditions. Clinical and laboratory studies in isolation units do not show a clear decrease in wound sepsis [4-41, 4-42]. Prevention of additional exogenous contamination seems to be important, however, and may be a factor in the ultimate healing of contaminated wounds [4-43].

Local Wound Care

Proper local treatment of the incised or accidentally inflicted wound has long been recognized as an important factor in the prevention of wound infection. Adequate and thorough debridement with removal of devitalized tissues is the most important deterrent to colonization by all forms of bacteria, including Clostridium, and especially *C. tetani.* [4-44]. The presence of avascular tissue or foreign bodies may allow a subinfective inoculum to produce wound sepsis [4-43, 4-45]. Interference with local blood supply has been shown to enhance bacterial growth [4-46] and even mild transient hemodynamic shock can allow invasive infection to occur [4-47]. The use of monofilament suture material may improve wound healing and not cause the same enhancement of infection as other materials [4-48].

Metabolic State of the Host

The general metabolic competence of the patient is clearly of importance. Wound infections occur more commonly in older patients and in patients with diabetes, obesity, malnutrition, or who are receiving steroid therapy [4-49]. Systemic trauma increases the chance of wound infection [4-50].

Antibody-Complement Interaction

Abnormalities of antibody synthesis may occur on a hereditary or acquired basis. Deficiencies in complement which occur in surgical patients are usually acquired and most often are secondary to massive injury, infection, and tissue damage [4-51, 4-52].

Impaired Perfusion

Phagocytic cells may not reach a contaminated focus due to defects in local or systemic circulation.

Neutrophils and Macrophages

Abnormalities of phagocytic cells may occur, neutrophils may be decreased or absent, or the ability of the neutrophils to kill ingested bacteria may be decreased [4-53]. A specific decrease in lysosomal enzymes of the neutrophil has been documented in patients with severe burns [4-54]. In addition, cyclic alterations in both phagocytosis and intracellular killing by neutrophils have been demonstrated [4-55]. The fixed macrophages of the reticulo-endothelial system may be depressed in function [4-56].

Factors involved in infections in surgical wounds were studied in a series of 15,000 patients in five different hospitals [4-57]. There was a positive correlation of wound infection with the degree of bacterial contamination, with the age of the patient, with the duration of the operative procedure, and with metabolic disturbances including diabetes, obesity, malnutrition, and previous steroid therapy. Long duration of preoperative hospitalization also seemed to increase the percentage of wound infection, a relationship not explained on the basis of other factors involved. Of considerable interest in this report was the great variability in incidence of infection among the hospitals studied, a difference not explained by the factors evaluated in the study. Within each hospital the various factors mentioned were important. However, one of the five hospitals maintained infection rates consistently lower than those of the other four, whereas one hospital maintained rates that were consistently higher. No explanation of this discrepancy could be found. It would appear that there are factors which affect postoperative wound infections that are not as yet measurable.

Antibiotics

The appropriate place of antibiotic agents in the prevention and treatment of wound infection has been debated for many years. It is clear that proper surgical drainage and debridement are always needed, and that appropriate antibiotics should be used when infection is present. Much discussion has centered upon the prophylactic use of antibiotics in the prevention of surgical wound infection. The use of prophylactic antibiotics has become an accepted principle in four major situations: (1) protection of healthy individuals against specific organisms, as the use of penicillin-G for prevention of gonorrhea or for the prevention of spread of meningococcal infections; (2) protection of acute or chronically ill individuals from secondary invesion, predominantly in the respiratory tract; (3) protection of a patient against the spread of a known infection, as in the drainage of large abscesses or in surgery in a patient with tuberculosis; and (4) protection of patients recovering from trauma or surgical operation when there is a recognized increased risk of infection. General guidelines for the use of prophylactic antibiotics suggest that high dosage and short period of administration are important, to prevent the development of resistant bacterial strains, and to keep from obscuring actual developing infection. Prophylactic antibiotics are considered justified when surgery must invade potentially contaminated organs such as the intestinal tract, when infectious processes such as abscesses are treated by surgical procedures, when contaminated wounds due to trauma must be treated, and in certain circumstances where infection is fraught with serious or fatal potential, as in cardiac and vascular operations where prostheses are used [4-58, 4-59].

PREOPERATIVE CARE

Preoperative preparation of the patient's skin requires optimization of the patient's general condition and restoration of the condition of the skin to normal. Infections must be treated and cleared, chronic skin conditions brought into the best possible condition, and, in the case of traumatic wounds, dirt and grease removed as thoroughly as possible.

INTRAOPERATIVE CARE

Intraoperative care requires thorough debridement of traumatic wounds, removal of devitalized tissues, gentle tissue handling, appropriate wound closure so as to minimize tissue damage and avoid deadspace and necrosis, and general support of the patient to maintain an optimum metabolic state. Wound closure should be complete whenever possible to allow physiologic sealing of the wound edges. Drains, tubes, and other foreign bodies which traverse the skin should be used only on specific indication.

POSTOPERATIVE CARE

In the *postoperative period* wound care requires daily inspection, exposure of the wound to its normal air environment whenever possible, and meticulous isolation in handling drains, tubes, and other transdermal foreign bodies. The use of local antibiotic ointment at the point of entry of such foreign bodies seems to be advisable.

REFERENCES

4-1.   Odland, G. F.: The Skin. Univ. of Washington School of Medicine, 1970.

4-2. Matoltsy, A. G.: What is keratin? In Advances in biology of skin, Vol. IX. New York, Pergamon Press, pp. 559–569.

4-3. Blank, I. H.: Factors which influence the water content of the stratum corneum. J. Invest. Derm. 18:433, 1952.

4-4. Scheuplein, R. J., and Morgan, L. J.: "Bound water" in keratin membranes measured by a microbalance technique. Nature 214: 456, 1967.

4-5. Blank, I. H., and Scheuplein, R. J.: Transport into and within the skin. Brit. J. Derm. 81 (Suppl. 4):4, 1969.

4-6. Middleton, J. D.: Pathways of penetration of electrolyte through stratum corneum. Brit. J. Derm. 81 (Suppl. 4):56, 1969.

4-7. Ross, R.: The fibroblast and wound repair. Biol. Rev. 43:51, 1968.

4-8. Kenede, R. M., Gibson, T., and Daly, C. H.: Bioengineering studies of the human skin. Symposium on Biomechanics and Related Bioengineering Topics. New York, Pergamon, 1965, pp. 147–158.

4-9. Ross, R., and Bornstein, P.: The elastic fiber. I. The separation and partial characterization of its macromolecular components. J. Cell Biol. 40:366, 1969.

4-10. Burton, A. C.: The physiology of cutaneous circulation, thermoregulatory functions. In Ed. Rothman, S. The Human Integument, Am. Asso. Adv. Sci; Wash. D.C. 1959, pp. 77–89.

4-11. Horstmann, E.: The lymph vessels of the skin. Die Ernalirung 68: 379, 1966.

4-12. Fox, R. H., and Edholm, O. G.: Nervous control of the cutaneous circulation. Brit. Med. Bull. 19:110, 1963.

4-13. Hertzman, A. B.: Vasomotor regulation of cutaneous circulation. Physiol. Rev. 39:280, 1959.

4-14. Cage, G. W., and Dobson, R. L.: Sodium secretion and reabsorption in the human eccrine sweat gland. J. Clin. Invest. 44:1270, 1965.

4-15. Brengelman, G., and Brown, A. C.: Temperature regulation. In Ruch, T. C., and Patton, H. D. (eds.): Physiology and Biophysics, 19th ed., Philadelphia, Saunders, 1965.

4-16. Burke, J. F., and Miles, A. A.: The sequence of vascular events in early infective inflammation. J. Path. Bact. 76:1, 1958.

4-17. Majno, G., and Palade, G. E.: Studies on inflammation. I. The effect of histamine and serotonin on vascular permeability: an electron microscopic study. J. Biophys. Biochem. Cytol. 11:571, 1961.

4-18. Border, J. R., Galo, E., and Schenk, W. G., Jr.: Systemic arteriovenous shunts in patients under severe stress: A common cause of high-output cardiac failure? Surgery 60:225, 1966.

4-19. Harrison, H. N., Moncrief, J. A., Duckett, J. W., Jr., and Mason, A. D. Jr:. The relationship between energy metabolism and water loss from vaporization in severely burned patients. Surgery 56:203, 1964.

4-20. Gump, F. E., Price, J. B., Jr., and Kinney, J. M.: Blood flow and oxygen consumption in patients with severe burns. Surg. Gynec. Obst. 130:23, 1970.

4-21. Roe, C. F., Kinney, J. M., and Blair, C.: Water and heat exchange in third degree burns. Surgery 56:212, 1964.

4-22. Jelenko, C., III, Wheeler, M. L., and Anderson, A. P.: The effect of topical sulfamylon on water loss through burn eschar: a re-evaluation. J. Trauma 10:1123, 1970.

4-23. Moser, M. H., Robinson, D. W., and Schloerb, P. R.: Transfers of water and electrolytes across granulation tissue in patients following burns. Surg. Gynec. Obst. 118:984, 1964.

4-24. Wilson, R. D., Knapp, C., Priano, L. L., and Traver, D. L.: Thermoregulatory failure of the burn scar. J. Trauma 11:518, 1971.

4-25. Jelenko, C., III, and Buxton, R. W.: The caloric significance of postburn surface water loss. Surgery 62:994, 1967.

4-26. Caldwell, F. T., Jr., and Levitsky, K.: Nitrogen balance after thermal burns. Effect of early eschar excision. Arch. Surg. 86:170, 1963.

4-27. Peacock, E. E., Jr., and Van Winkle, W., Jr.: Surgery and biology of wound repair. Philadelphia, Saunders, 1970, pp. 41–42.

4-28. Johnson, F. R.: The reaction of the epithelium to injury. Sci. Basis Med. Ann. Rev., 1964, pp. 276–290.

4-29. Madden, J. W., and Peacock, E. E., Jr.: Studies on the biology of collagen during wound healing. I. Rate of collagen synthesis and deposition in cutaneous wounds of the rat. Surgery 64:288, 1968.

4-30. Peacock, E. E., Jr., and Van Winkle, W., Jr.: Surgery and biology of wound repair. Philadelphia, Saunders, 1970, pp. 167–168.

4-31. Stephens, F. O., and Hunt, T. K.: Effect of changes in inspired oxygen and carbon dioxide tensions on wound tensile strength: An experimental study. Ann. Surg. 173:515, 1971.

4-32. Donati, R. M., Frank, D. W., Stromberg, L. R., and McLaughlin, M. M.: The effect of the germ-free state on wound healing. J. Surg. Res. 11:163, 1971.

4-33. Cole, W. R., and Bernard, H. R.: Inadequacies of present methods of surgical skin preparation. Arch. Surg. 89:215, 1964.

4-34. Dineen, P.: An evaluation of the duration of the surgical scrub. Surg. Gynec. Obst. 129:1181, 1969.

4-35. Carpendale, M. T. F., and Sereda, W.: The role of the percutaneous suture in surgical wound infection. Surgery 58:672, 1965.

4-36. Schauerhamer, R. A., Edlich, R. F., Panek, P., Thul, J., Prusak, M., and Wangensteen, O. H.: Studies in the management of the contaminated wound. VII. Susceptibility of surgical wounds to postoperative surface contamination. Am. J. Surg. 122:74, 1971.

4-37. Fuchs, P. C.: Indwelling intravenous polyethylene catheters: factors influencing the risk of microbial colonization and sepsis. JAMA 216:1447, 1971.

4-38.   Bernard, R. W., Stahl, W. M., and Chase, R. M., Jr.: Subclavian Vein Catheterizations: A Prospective Study: II, Infectious Complications. Ann. Surg. 173:191, 1971.

4-39.   Barclay, T. L., and Dexter, F.: Infection and cross-infection in a new burns centre. Brit. J. Surg. 55:197, 1968.

4-40.   Sutter, V. L., and Hurst, V.: Sources of *Pseudomonas aeruginosa* infection in burns: Study of wound and rectal cultures with phage typing. Ann. Surg. 163:597, 1966.

4-41.   Nance, F. C., Lewis, V., and Bornside, G. H.: Absolute barrier isolation and antibiotics in the treatment of experimental burn wound sepsis. J. Surg. Res. 10:33, 1970.

4-42.   Haynes, B. W., Jr.: Patient isolation and patient isolators. J. Trauma 7:95, 1967.

4-43.   Howe, C. W.: Experimental studies on determinants of wound infection. Surg. Gynec. Obst. 123:507, 1966.

4-44.   Altemeier, W. A., and Hummel, R. P.: Treatment of tetanus. Surgery 60:495, 1966.

4-45.   Elek, S. D., and Conen, P. E.: The virulence of staphylococcus pyogenes for man. A study of the problems of wound infection. Brit. J. Exp. Path. 38:573, 1957.

4-46.   Miles, A. A., Miles, E. M., and Burke, J.: The value and duration of defence reactions of the skin to the primary lodgement of bacteria. Brit. J. Exp. Path. 38:79, 1957.

4-47.   DeWitt, R. J., and Stahl, W. M.: Lymphatic flora in third degree burns. Surg. Forum 15:41, 1964.

4-48.   Ferguson, D. J.: Clinical application of experimental relations between technique and wound infection. Surgery 63:377, 1968.

4-49.   Stephens, F. O., Hunt, T. K., Jawetz, E., Sonne, M., and Dunphy, J. E.: Effect of cortisone and vitamin A on wound infection. Am. J. Surg. 121:569, 1971.

4-50.   Conolly, W. B., Hunt, T. K., Sonne, M., and Dunphy, J. E.: Influence of distant trauma on local wound infection. Surg. Gynec. Obst. 128:713, 1969.

4-51.   Feingold, D. S.: Hospital-acquired infections. New Engl. J. Med. 283:1384, 1970.

4-52.   Alexander, J. W., and Moncrief, J. A.: Alterations of the immune response following severe thermal injury. Arch. Surg. 93:75, 1966.

4-53.   Alexander, J. W., and Fisher, M. W. Immunological determinants of pseudomonas infections of man accompanying severe burn injury. J. Trauma 10:565, 1970.

4-54.   Alexander, J. W.: Serum and leukocyte lysosomal enzyme derangements following severe thermal injury. Arch. Surg. 95:482, 1967.

4-55.   Alexander, J. W.: Surgical infections—pathogen versus host. J. Surg. Res. 8:225, 1968.

4-56.   Alexander, J. W., and Meakins, J. L.: Natural defense mechanisms
        in clinical sepsis. J. Surg. Res. 11:148, 1971.
4-57.   Report of an Ad Hoc Committee on Trauma: Postoperative Wound
        Infections. Ann. Surg. 160: (Suppl.) 1–192, 1964.
4-58.   Altemeier, W. A., Barnes, B. A., Pulaski, E. J., Sandusky, W. R.,
        Burke, J. F., and Clowes, G. H. A., Jr.: Infections: Prophylaxis
        and management—a symposium. Surgery 67:369, 1970.
4-59.   Moore, W. S., Rosson, C. T., and Hall, A. D.: Effect of prophylactic
        antibiotics in preventing bacteremic infection of vascular pros-
        theses. Surgery 69:825, 1971.

PART II

Transport Systems

5

CARDIOVASCULAR SYSTEM

GENERAL FUNCTION

The cardiovascular system consists of a muscular pump, the heart, and two systems of branching arteries, capillaries, and veins, which allow blood to flow through the lungs and through the body tissues. The function of this system is to provide sufficient flow to the pulmonary bed to allow for gas exchange, and to provide adequate flow to peripheral tissues for the delivery of fuel for cell metabolic needs and the removal of products of metabolism.

The heart must provide an adequate minute output to accomplish these needs at rest, and must be able to respond to any normal increase in the level of body-tissue metabolism. Normal function of the heart as a muscular pump depends upon the strength and velocity of cardiac muscle contraction. All ventricular muscle fibers must contract simultaneously, and the rhythmic sequence of such contraction must be appropriate to allow proper filling and emptying of the cardiac chambers. The cardiac valves must function adequately without significant stenosis or regurgitation. Abnormal shunts must not exist between the pulmonary and systemic circulations.

PHYSIOLOGY OF CONTRACTION

Cardiac Muscle-Cell Organization

The ventricular myocardium is composed of striated muscle cells, 10 to 15 millimicrons ($m\mu$) in diameter, and 30 to 60 $m\mu$ in length. Each cell contains multiple cross-banded myofibrils which run the length of the cell. These myofibrils in turn are composed of groups of myofilaments aligned parallel to give the whole fiber its banded appearance [5-1]. Interactions between the myofilaments provide the shortening of cardiac muscle contracture. The remainder of the cell cytoplasm contains the other cell constituents, including the nucleus and the usual cell organelles.

The myocardial fibers branch and interdigitate with one another. A special portion of the sarcolemma or cell membrane, the intercalated disc, joins these fiber branches to produce a continuous mesh [5-2]. The low electrical resistance of the intercalated disc allows for the spread of excitation and the transmission of contraction across the muscle fibers [5-3].

Cell Energy

Mitochondria form approximately 25 to 30 per cent of the entire cell mass of the fiber. The release of energy from body fuel is accomplished within the mitochondria by oxidative phosphorylation to produce adenosine triphosphate (ATP). This ATP then provides energy for contraction of the myofibrils. The large numbers of mitochondria in cardiac muscle cells indicate the high energy requirement for cardiac function.

Fibril Contraction

Each segment of the cardiac muscle fiber (sarcomere) is composed of two sets of myofilaments; a thick filament composed of myosin, and a thinner filament composed of actin. These two types of myofilament are arranged in parallel ranks with overlapping of ranks of the thick and thin filaments [5-4, 5-5]. Muscular contraction occurs due to sliding of these ranks of filaments into closer apposition. Both thick and thin contractile filaments remain constant in overall length, whether at rest or during contraction [5-6]. The movement of the alternating sets of myofibrils to produce contraction appears to be caused by interaction of the filaments in such a way as to produce directional forces which close the ranks of the long fibrils without altering fibril length.

During this contraction, linkages are made between actin and myosin filaments which are broken during relaxation. During contraction ATP is split by a magnesium activated ATPase which requires trace amounts of calcium [5-7]. The small amounts of calcium required to regulate this reaction appear to be cyclically released and reaccumulated by the longitudinal sarcoplasmic reticulum.

The reticulum is a series of longitudinal interconnecting tubules closely applied to the surfaces of the individual segments of the myofibers. At the end of each segment, the longitudinal tubular systems coalesce to form a cistern which has been shown in vitro to have the ability to accumulate calcium from the surrounding solution [5-8]. The sarcoplasmic reticulum appears also to be able to transmit an action potential to all areas of the sarcomere. This reticulum thus seems to be an important factor in the excitation of cardiac muscle contraction [5-9].

Basis for Starling's Law of the Heart

A basic pattern of function of heart muscle is the relationship between initial muscle length and the ability to develop force, termed Starling's Law of the Heart. This law states that an increase in initial ventricular volume results in an increase in the force of ventricular contraction [5-10, 5-11]. The length of the sarcomere, representing the degree of overlapping of the ranks of myosin and actin fibrils, is directly proportional to cardiac muscle length [5-12]. This is also true for skeletal muscle [5-13]. Ultrastructural studies have shown that the degree of interdigitation of adjoining ranks of myosin and actin fibrils is the basis for Starling's Law of the Heart. From a position of maximal overlap (contracture) increase in muscle length provides a larger surface between actin and myosin fibers, thus producing increasing contractile ability. Stretch of the muscle beyond an optimal point (L_{max}) distracts adjacent ranks of fibrils and areas of overlap decrease, producing a gradual fall of contractile ability to zero with maximum stretch [5-14].

Force-Velocity Relationships

The force of contracture of cardiac muscle fibers and the rapidity of shortening of these fibers determines the ability of the intact heart to function as a pump. The force-velocity relationships are controlled in two ways: The first is by the Frank-Starling mechanism, apparently due to the increase in the number of contractile sites of myosin and actin which are apposed to each other as fiber length increases. This mechanism provides for an increase in maximum isometric force with increasing initial muscle length with no change in the maximal velocity of shortening [5-15]. A second method for altering the force-velocity relationship is by inotropic alteration. This produces an increase in the maximum velocity of fiber shortening (V_{max}), apparently by increasing the force generated at each contractile site. Norepinephrine, calcium, digitalis glycosides, increasing frequency of contraction, and sustained postextrasystolic potentiation (paired electrical stimulation), produce an increase in V_{max} with or without a change in maximum isometric force (P_0) [5-16, 5-17, 5-18, 5-19].

Measurement of the rate of force development (dp/dt) is a measure of the force-velocity ratio of heart muscle and depends on the P_0 and the V_{max} of the muscle fibers. This measurement is made during the isometric contraction period. This is important since the actual force developed is influenced by the elastic elements of the muscle fiber and by the degree of afterload, factors which are minimized during contraction around a stable volume.

CARDIAC FUNCTION

Systemic Influences

In the intact animal and man humoral and reflex factors influence cardiac function and at times may overshadow the Frank-Starling mechanism. Changes in myocardial contractility, heart rate, venous return, and peripheral vascular resistance due to humoral and neural influences are present in almost every acute change of state.

Ventricular Function Curves

The function of the intact heart as a pump has been studied by relating cardiac filling pressure or ventricular end diastolic pressure to stroke work. It is thus possible to construct ventricular function curves [5-20]. Cardiac work is plotted upward on the ordinate, with filling pressure plotted to the right on the abcissa. Improved performance with increase in work output at normal filling pressures results in "elevation" of the function curve. With a decrease in cardiac performance, normal work is accomplished only at higher filling pressures, and the curve is depressed and moved to the right.

Adrenergic Stimulation

The effect of adrenergic stimulation on myocardial performance has long been known. Stimulation of local norepinephrine release results in an elevation (improvement) of the ventricular-function curve. The effects produced are an increase in heart rate, a reduction in ventricular volume, an increase in the rate of development of pressure, and an increase in the velocity of ejection [5-21, 5-22].

Cholinergic Stimulation

Vagal stimulation may have a negative inotropic effect on left ventricular contraction [5-23], and has a definite negative inotropic effect on atrial contraction and atrioventricular conduction.

Denervation

Studies of the denervated heart indicate that the intrinsic contractile properties are maintained, and cardiac function can still rise to meet the demands for energy [5-24, 5-25]. Under these circumstances, the Frank-Starling mechanism increases stroke volume and cardiac output with little increase in heart rate.

Rhythm Effects

Another factor influencing the strength of ventricular contraction is the time relationship between subsequent beats. Premature depolarization and contraction results in reduced contractile force while the subsequent contraction is more forceful than normal. This augmentation of myocardial contractility following extrasystole has been used to increase myocardial force (paired electrical stimulation) [5-26, 5-27].

MYOCARDIAL OXYGEN REQUIREMENTS

Pressure/Volume Influences

Myocardial oxygen consumption appears to be most directly related to the level of pressure required (aortic pressure) as transmitted by tension of the myocardial fiber, and the speed with which this tension is achieved, the so-called time-tension index. It has been known for many years that "pressure work" requires more oxygen consumption than does "volume work," and increases in stroke volume without increases in the afterloading pressure require very small increments in oxygen consumption [5-28]. Increase in the velocity of contraction (V_{max}) has been shown to increase oxygen need even when the time-tension index is reduced [5-29, 5-30].

Myocardial Anoxia

The source of energy for contraction of myocardial fibers is ATP formed by oxidative phosphorylation of substrate. Under normal conditions glucose, fatty acids, lactate, pyruvate, acetate, ketone bodies, and amino acids can serve as energy sources [5-31]. The production of myocardial anoxia with a shift to anaerobic metabolism markedly reduces the effectiveness of phosphorylation, and a fall in ventricular performance has been noted in experimental models when anoxia is produced [5-32].

REGULATION OF CARDIAC OUTPUT

Guyton has stressed the importance of oxygen delivery and utilization by the cell as the primary factor in the regulation of local tissue vascular resistance and thus in regulation of cardiac output. He has pointed out that tissue metabolism suffers due to anoxia if cardiac output is reduced to two-thirds of normal—although glucose, amino acids, fat, and other nutriments are delivered to the peripheral tissues in completely adequate amounts at a much lower cardiac output. Removal of carbon dioxide, lactic acid, and other metabolic products also is accomplished at a much lower level of cardiac output [5-33].

Tissue Hypoxia

Tissue hypoxia produces local vasodilatation. This vasodilatation occurs in response to local metabolic factors, either from relaxation of smooth muscle due directly to the lack of oxygen or from the release of local vasodilator materials. It occurs immediately upon perfusion of vessels with hypoxemic blood and is not dependent upon sympathetic innervation [5-34, 5-35].

As vasodilatation occurs in local tissue beds, total peripheral vascular resistance is decreased. Systemic blood pressure decreases enough to stimulate the carotid and aortic pressure receptors. Sympathetic activity is stimulated, with direct effect on myocardial norepinephrine release. Vasoconstriction of other vascular beds is produced, and adrenal medullary release of catecholamines is stimulated. Simultaneously venous return increases. These factors combine to increase cardiac output. Cardiac output, therefore, increases in response to a decrease in atmospheric oxygen concentration [5-36], to a lowering of the oxygen content of circulating blood [5-37], and to a reduction in the ability of the tissue cells to utilize oxygen [5-38].

Exercise

Reduction in vascular resistance in skeletal muscle beds occurs during muscular exercise due to the sudden increase in metabolic activity. Cardiac output may rise manyfold to meet these demands [5-39, 5-40].

Inflammation

Increase in cardiac output results from the decrease in local vascular resistance caused by inflammation. Such increases occur in patients with severe infections due to increased blood flow through the infected areas [5-41]. Higher levels of cardiac output are also seen in patients with widespread skin damage due to burns, presumably due to greater volume of cutaneous blood flow [5-42]. Increase in cardiac output occurs in certain patients with septic shock, where lowered peripheral resistance results from failure of cell utilization of oxygen [5-43, 5-44], and in certain conditions where humoral agents depress peripheral vasoconstriction, exemplified by the hyperdynamic state found in certain cirrhotic patients [5-45].

Mechanisms of Cardiac-Output Response

The heart can increase cardiac output by two basic mechanisms—an increase in cardiac rate, and an increase in stroke volume. In addition, autonomic stimulation and inotropic agents can alter the performance curve of cardiac contraction to increase V_{max} and shorten systolic ejection time for a given ventricular volume. All of these mechanisms come into play in the conditions described. Moderate exercise has been shown to cause an increase in heart rate and an increase in ventricular contractility [5-46] with only a small increase in stroke volume. With increasing exertion, stroke volume can increase as much as 100 per cent [5-47]. Increase in the stroke volume is accomplished by the operation of the Frank-Starling law, and is capable of responding to the demands of exercise even in the presence of cardiac denervation and adrenalectomy [5-21]. Increase in cardiac rate above 120 to 130/min shortens cardiac filling time and results in a progressive decrease in cardiac output [5-14, 5-48]. Changes in cardiac rate and cardiac contractility appear to be due to activity of the sympathetic nervous system [5-49], while stroke volume changes appear to be due to increased venous return.

CARDIAC FAILURE

Failure of the heart to maintain a cardiac output sufficient for metabolic demand occurs under a variety of conditions. Primary cardiac disease, either myocardial or valvular, frequently results in cardiac failure. Inability of the heart to maintain adequate output is the eventual cause of death in a variety of forms of shock.

Decrease in Myocardial Work

The pathophysiology of cardiac failure has been intensively studied. Cardiac failure is characterized by a decrease in the external work of the myocardium, although oxygen uptake remains the same [5-14]. Tissue analysis for high-energy phosphates reveals no deficit, and energy liberation by analysis of the breakdown of ATP is apparently normal. Myocardial contractility, however, is depressed, with reduction of V_{max} and reduction in the maximum isometric tension that can be achieved (P_0) [5-50]. This alteration is caused by a depression both in the velocity and in the extent of myocardial fiber shortening in congestive heart failure [5-51]. Thus, the failing heart delivers a smaller than normal volume from a normal or elevated end diastolic volume, a change recognized as early as 1914 [5-23].

Studies of norepinephrine concentrations in myocardial tissues of both animals and man in cardiac failure have shown marked depletion of such stores [5-52, 5-53]. This is apparently due to a decrease in norepinephrine biosynthesis, since tyrosine hydroxylase activity is also reduced.

Increase in Heart Rate

In the intact animal, compensatory mechanisms come into play when myocardial contractility is reduced. Heart rate increases, presumably as a result of sympathetic activity. This increase in rate enables the heart to maintain the cardiac output at a reduced stroke volume, and there may actually be a decrease in resistance to cardiac ejection at the more rapid rate [5-54].

Increase in End Diastolic Volume

As stroke volume increases, the end diastolic volume increases and cardiac dilatation takes place. This permits the ejection of an adequate stroke volume even with reduced contractility of the myocardial elements. With the patient at rest, cardiac output and stroke volume may be normal. The ratio of the stroke volume to end diastolic volume is depressed, however [5-55]. Left ventricular performance as evaluated by the response to exercise shows that left ventricular end diastolic pressure rises in the patient with heart failure. Likewise, the rate of systolic ejection is depressed both at rest and following exercise [5-56].

Increase in End Diastolic Pressure

Maintenance of a normal cardiac output under conditions of cardiac failure is achieved only with an elevation of the ventricular end diastolic pressure.

Dyspnea and Pulmonary Edema

Elevation of left ventricular end diastolic pressure increases pulmonary capillary pressure with the resulting danger of pulmonary edema. As myocardial contractility decreases this effect is intensified. Pulmonary capillaries become engorged, and interstitial and alveolar edema may be produced. Dyspnea and tachypnea occur, apparently due to stimulation of vagal stretch receptors [5-57].

Generalized Fluid Retention

Fluid retention occurs due to the increase in systemic venous pressure produced by the rise in right ventricular end diastolic pressure, and because of the renal effects of decreased cardiac output. Proximal tubular resorption of sodium is enhanced by decreased renal blood flow, and distal tubular resorption is increased by the stimulation of the renin-aldosterone mechanism. Elevation of renal venous pressure also increases sodium retention. While some degree of increase in total blood volume may aid the failing heart due to improved cardiac filling, further expansion exaggerates the increased venous pressure and produces further myocardial overload.

Increased Oxygen Extraction by Tissues

With restriction of the cardiac output, peripheral tissue oxygen needs can be met for a time by an increase in oxygen extraction from circulating blood. The A-V oxygen difference increases and P_vO_2 falls. Anaerobic metabolism with the production of lactic acidemia occurs when this compensatory mechanism fails to provide adequate minute oxygen delivery to tissue cells.

Cardiogenic Shock

The point at which all compensatory mechanisms fail to provide cell oxygenation adequate for metabolic needs defines the onset of cardiogenic shock. Congestive failure may exist for long periods of time as long as the low cardiac output and all compensating changes provide sufficient oxygen delivery for basal metabolism. A fall in cardiac output below this level, whether acutely induced or occurring during the course of congestive failure, produces cell anoxia and progressive acidosis, a condition leading to death unless reversible by therapy. Such a degree of failure of myocardial performance is usually associated with severe myocardial damage [5-58].

EFFECTS OF STRESS STATES ON CARDIAC OUTPUT

The increase in metabolic demand produced by surgery, trauma, and infection, requires an appropriate response in cardiac performance. Shoemaker and co-workers have characterized the changes in demand for cardiac output which result from injury, hemorrhage, and infection [5-59].

Hemorrhage

In acute hemorrhage with hypovolemic shock, venous return to the heart is decreased and there is a low cardiac output and a low stroke volume. Compensation occurs by increasing heart rate and by increasing peripheral vascular resistance. Vasoconstriction in splanchnic, renal, and dermal vasculature redistributes blood from the central core and skin. This works to maintain blood pressure, and to preserve flow to brain and heart.

Trauma

Unanesthetized trauma results in an increase in cardiac output with an increase in both heart rate and stroke volume. In these patients autonomic drive appears to be increased and peripheral resistance falls.

Effects of Anesthesia

Trauma which occurs under anesthesia is accompanied by a greater fall in blood pressure and a smaller rise in cardiac output than when no anesthesia is present. This change occurs at a slightly increased venous pressure. Peripheral resistance is decreased to a greater extent than in the unanesthetized state. Stroke volume and stroke work fall when trauma is sustained under anesthesia, whereas these functions rise in unanesthetized patients. All of these studies would suggest that anesthesia itself interferes with the maximal cardiac response to injury, perhaps by blocking the central nervous system diencephalic response due to the unconscious state of the patient, and perhaps by altering peripheral vascular reactivity and myocardial contractility.

Sepsis

Patients in septic shock characteristically have an elevated cardiac output with low peripheral resistance. Oxygen consumption is usually decreased, indicating a block at the cellular level [5-60].

Acidosis

The effect of acidosis on myocardial function is not clear. Experimental studies have failed to show a consistent decrease in cardiac contractility with the production of acidosis [5-61, 5-62, 5-63], and some authors have shown an increase in cardiac function [5-64]. A decrease in the response to injected norepinephrine has also been seen [5-65]. It has been shown that a decrease in pH markedly effects the function of guinea pig atrial muscle in vitro after depletion of catecholamine [5-66]. Clinically, the acidotic state increases the incidence of cardiac arrhythmias.

Terminal Failure of Cardiac Performance

Demise of the patient from any form of shock occurs when hemodynamic decompensation takes place. This may take the form of a fall in peripheral resistance with hypotension, cardiac failure with elevated central venous pressure, low cardiac output, bradycardia and arrhythmias, maldistribution of blood flow and blood volume, and severe metabolic alterations.

Carey and co-workers noted that in chronically stressed patients the cardiac output rose primarily due to changes in heart rate and myocardial contractility. However, heart rate usually leveled off at 100 to 120 beats/min, and further increases were produced by increase in stroke volume [5-60]. Their studies suggested a stabilization of the autonomic control mechanisms at a maximal level, with an increasing role played by the Frank-Starling mechanism as cardiac output demands increased. It may be that in the state of prolonged stress, myocardial norepinephrine stores are depleted, a condition analagous to that which occurs in the failing heart. The suggestion has also been made that a specific myocardial depressant factor is produced by prolonged shock and sepsis [5-67, 5-68]. This factor seems to arise from the anoxic splanchnic tissues [5-69, 5-70] and may be removed by hemodialysis [5-71].

ASSESSMENT OF CARDIAC FUNCTION

The adequacy of function of the cardiovascular system is measured by the ability of the heart to provide circulation appropriate to the metabolic demands of the tissues. A first line of measurement, therefore, is a careful analysis of the hemodynamic status of the patient at rest.

General Appearance

General appraisal of the patient's condition should be made with special attention to signs of tissue anoxia and/or excessive sympathetic tone. These include restlessness progressing to coma, dyspnea and tachypnea, skin pallor, coolness, and the production of sweat.

Heart Rate and Rhythm

Measurement of the heart rate and determination of the exact rhythm must be done. Serious arrhythmias interfere with cardiac filling and ejection. A heart rate below 40/min may deliver an inadequate cardiac output, even at large stroke volumes, while a heart rate over 120/min may be too rapid to allow adequate cardiac filling. Tachycardia above 100/min may be a compensation for inadequate myocardial contractility. The adequacy of the pulse pressure is important as a measurement both of myocardial performance and of the degree of peripheral vasoconstriction. A decrease in myocardial contractility or a severe increase in generalized vasomotor tone will decrease the pulse pressure.

Renal Function

Renal function responds dramatically to changes in cardiac output. Conditions of this response are the preexistence of relatively adequate renal function and the absence of diuretic activity from administered drug or endogenous hyperglycemia. With fall in cardiac output, proximal tubular resorption of sodium increases, and distal tubular resorption of sodium and water is enhanced. Oliguria or anuria results with the production of a very concentrated urine. An hourly urine output of 30 to 50 ml/min in the 70 kg adult who is not dehydrated is indicative of adequate cardiac output.

Central Venous Pressure

Measurement of right ventricular filling pressure (right atrial pressure) adds another dimension to the assessment of cardiac function. The comparison of assessment of the effects of cardiac activity and the filling pressure at which these effects are achieved is a rough ventricular function curve. Signs of inadequate cardiac output and an elevation of the right atrial pressure above 12 to 14 cm H_2O indicate poor cardiac performance, whereas the reverse—i.e., a normal (5 to 12 cm H_2O) right atrial pressure in the presence of evidence of adequate tissue perfusion—indicates cardiac output adequate for the state of the patient at the time of measurement. Central venous pressure is less accurate in measuring elevations of left atrial pressure. However, pulmonary artery pressure may reveal early left ventricular failure [5-72]. Pulmonary capillary wedged pressure is more closely correlated to left ventricular performance [5-73].

Blood Gas Analysis

The use of blood-gas measurements and the assessment of the acid-base balance of the patient is of vital importance in determining whether tissue perfusion is adequate for metabolic needs. If perfusion falls, the first response is an increased extraction of oxygen from the flowing blood. Measurement of arterial and venous gases will show an increased A-V oxygen difference caused by a low mixed venous P_{O_2}. This "poor man's cardiac output" is only relatively accurate. However, a mixed venous P_{O_2} persistently below 25 is almost always a sign of severe depression of cardiac output and eventual demise from this cause alone. If tissue anoxia occurs in spite of increased oxygen extraction, lactic acidemia results with a fall in blood pH. The normal compensation for this metabolic acidosis is hyperventilation with a reduction in the P_{CO_2} to bring pH values toward normal. It is therefore necessary to measure pH, P_{CO_2}, and P_{O_2} in arterial and venous blood to make the appropriate determination of oxygen extraction and acid-base profile. Levels of excess lactate can be measured independently.

The assessment described can be done at the bedside at frequent intervals [5-74]. With the exception of the central venous pressure (right atrial pressure), all of the factors in this assessment pertain to a rough evaluation of the adequacy of tissue perfusion. Right-atrial pressure measurements give a rough indication of the adequacy of myocardial function in its production of this perfusion state. None of these measurements indicate the competence of myocardial contractility or the normality of chamber filling and cardiac ejection. The reserve ability of the heart to respond to increased demands of tissue metabolism remains unknown.

Cardiac Reserve

In assessing cardiac reserve function, detection of abnormalities in valvular function by physical examination should be carefully done. A history of myocardial infarction, or evidence on electrocardiography of left bundle branch block, endocardial damage, previous myocardial infarction, left ventricular hypertrophy, or the presence of T-wave changes interpreted as left ventricular strain pattern all have been shown to be associated with diminished myocardial reserve. Such patients have an increased potential for myocardial infarction in the intra- and postoperative periods [5-75].

Exercise Test

An exercise test may be used to unmask myocardial insufficiency. Electrocardiographic changes following exercise and abnormal tachycardia or elevation of the right atrial pressure are signs of poor myocardial reserve. Increase in the A-V oxygen difference may also be seen following exercise in such patients.

Cardiac Output

Measurement of cardiac output can be done by a variety of means. Each method has certain inherent problems and inaccuracies and some are far more complex than others. The Fick principle states that if one knows the concentration of a substance before and after its passage through a tissue bed, and if one can measure the amount of new substance added or subtracted within that tissue bed one is able to calculate the rate of flow. In terms of cardiac output, this calculation is as follows: Total flow in ml/min is equal to the oxygen uptake in ml/min divided by the arteriovenous oxygen difference. This method requires arterial and venous sampling and precise measurement of oxygen uptake during a measured time.

The indicator dilution technique for measurement of blood flow is analogous to the Fick principle and is performed by the rapid injection of an indicator into the circulation and its measurement at some downstream sampling area. Indicator dilution methodology has been used most frequently with the dye, indocyanine green. Presently accepted methodology uses indocyanine green with right atrial injection and peripheral artery or central aorta sampling [5-76]. Although there may be variations between dye-dilution cardiac output studies and the cardiac output measured by direct electromagnetic techniques [5-77], repeated measurements with indocyanine green have been shown to correlate within 0.245 liters/min under controlled conditions [5-78].

Saline, radioactive materials, and hot and cold solutions (thermodilution) have also been used as indicators [5-79, 5-80, 5-81, 5-82, 5-83]. All of the indicator dilution techniques work with reasonable accuracy in states of normal cardiac output but show increasing inaccuracies with low flow and in situations of cardiopulmonary disease [5-77]. Calculation of the cardiac output by indicator dilution methods is usually made using the formula suggested by Stewart and modified by Hamilton [5-84].

Many attempts have been made to measure cardiac output by less complicated and less invasive techniques. Analysis of the pulse contour and pulse pressure has been suggested by Warner and associates as a method of determining cardiac output [5-85]. Comparison of the cardiac output as measured by analysis of the central aortic pulse contour and by simultaneous dye dilution determinations has shown agreement within 9 to 16 per cent [5-86, 5-87].

A completely noninvasive technique has been devised using electrical impedance measurements which vary depending upon the composition of the tissue through which the electric discharge must pass. Variations in fluid content, therefore, vary the impedance of the thorax. Impedance plethysmography has been used to measure cardiac output in man [5-88]. Studies using the impedance-plethysmography technique have shown reasonably good correlation with indicator dilution or pulse pressure methods in normal subjects [5-88] or in patients with chronic cardiac disease [5-89] studied in the erect position. The application of this technique to sick patients in the supine position, however, revealed poor quantitative correlation. Qualitative changes, however, were indicated [5-90].

Circulation Time

In addition to the measurement of cardiac output, the dye dilution technique allows measurement of circulation time and the calculation of central blood volume.

Myocardial Performance

A further use of the indicator dilution curve has been suggested by Goodwin et al. These workers calculated the residual ventricular volume from a portion of the standard dye curve. They showed that an enlarged end diastolic ventricular volume was associated with decreased cardiac reserve and with an increased risk of operation [5-91]. Measurement of the ventricular pressure curves has been used by Siegel et al to calculate an index of survival, relating ventricular reserve to peripheral resistance factors [5-92]. Pulse-contour techniques and thoracic impedance plethysmography have been used as a method of evaluating myocardial contractility [5-90, 5-93]. These techniques thus offer an additional way of assessing myocardial function.

PREOPERATIVE EVALUATION

History

The aim of the preoperative cardiovascular evaluation is to determine the state of the cardiovascular system at the time of assessment and to discover any factors which may indicate decreased cardiac reserve. A careful history of previous cardiac disease is of utmost importance. Preexisting damage inflicted on cardiac muscle through disease of the coronary arteries or defects due to any of the varieties of valvular disease clearly decrease functional reserve of the heart. The history should include an assessment of the present competence of the cardiovascular system of the patient. The ability of the patient to move about, climb stairs, and do work is clearly important.

Physical Examination

The physical examination should include a careful measurement of heart rate and rhythm; determination of skin color, texture, and turgor; palpation of pulses, and determination of obvious signs of venous engorgement. Heart size should be estimated and abnormal heart sounds sought. Auscultation of the lungs for any early pulmonary edema is important. Evaluation of liver size should be made. Funduscopic examination, auscultation of the carotid vessels, and palpation and auscultation of the vessels of the abdomen and extremities will give important information as to the state of the entire vascular system. The arterial blood pressure should be measured in more than one extremity. The legs and sacral areas should be examined for edema.

Laboratory Studies

Initial laboratory studies should include a chest x-ray, PA and lateral films, for determination of heart size and pulmonary or pleural pathology. The standard electrocardiogram should be obtained. The hematocrit should be measured and a white blood count obtained. Blood chemistries should be determined to assess the function of the liver and kidneys and to assure a normal electrolyte pattern.

Special Tests

If all of these usual measurements are normal and the patient has been carrying on an active life, the risk of major surgery of the usual magnitude is not significant from the point of view of the cardiovascular system and further studies are probably not indicated in the preoperative period. If, however, there is a history of cardiac disease or abnormality in the electrocardiogram, then an exercise tolerance test should be carried out, taking postexercise electrocardiographic tracings. Measurement of the central venous pressure in the postexercise period should be done. In addition, arterial and venous blood gases should be measured. In certain instances estimation of the left ventricular residual volume and measurement of left ventricular myocardial function should be performed.

PREOPERATIVE PREPARATION

The cardiovascular status of the patient should be optimized prior to the scheduled operation. This may mean regulation of digitalis dosage or the institution of digitalization. In the case of overt congestive failure, therapy with diuretics may be necessary. Arrhythmias should receive appropriate pharmacologic therapy, and serious conduction defects with slow ventricular rate may require the insertion of a transvenous pacemaker. Blood chemical abnormalities and any deficit in hematocrit should be corrected.

INTRAOPERATIVE CARE

Monitoring

Any patient undergoing a major operative procedure should have appropriate catheters inserted to allow measurement of urine output and central venous pressure during the procedure. Arterial pressure can, in most cases, be measured by the standard blood-pressure cuff. The patient should be monitored by continuous display of the electrocardiogram for constant observation of cardiac rate and rhythm. It should be emphasized that the normal appearance of the electrocardiographic tracing does not indicate adequate cardiac output [5-94]. Measurement of peripheral pulses and blood pressure and interval measurement of blood gases is the only way to prove the adequacy of perfusion. Normal electrocardiographic tracings may persist at times when myocardial contractility has been reduced by injected drugs and cardiac output is at dangerously low levels. The absence of detectable blood pressure and pulse indicate this failure of perfusion. Closed cardiac massage is mandatory under such circumstances, even in the presence of a normal electrocardiogram.

Anesthesia

The anesthesiologist should choose an anesthetic agent which does not depress myocardial function. Rapid-acting barbiturates should be watched closely in this regard. Excessive vasoconstriction should be avoided (cyclopropane). In general, anesthesia should be sufficient to render the patient amnesic, and relaxation should be obtained by the use of relaxant drugs.

Surgery

ABDOMINAL REFLEX CHANGES

The surgical technique used must be as atraumatic and gentle as possible, especially within the abdomen. It has been shown that reflex bradycardia and dilatation of peripheral vascular beds can occur following stimulation of the splanchnic organs [5-95]. Bradycardia appears to be caused by increased vagal tone and can be blocked by the administration of atropine. Dilatation of both capacitance and resistance vessels appears to be due to inhibition of tonic sympathetic activity. The result of these two effects is a dramatic fall in blood pressure, decrease in cardiac output, and decrease in tissue perfusion. In most cases cessation of the operative manipulation will permit restoration of heart rate and sympathetic tone to normal without therapy. If these undesired results recur on manipulation of the area, blockade of afferent nerve impulses with local anesthesia may be considered. It may be dangerous to attempt to restore blood pressure by rapid infusion of volume in such patients because overtransfusion may occur.

Hypotension

The occurrence of hypotension, due either to reflex stimulation or to unreplaced hypovolemia, is associated with an increased incidence of intra- and postoperative myocardial infarction [5-96]. Hypotension should be avoided whenever possible by gentleness in surgical technique and by concomitant replacement of any lost whole blood. Replacement of extracellular fluid losses should be made during major abdominal surgery by the use of Ringer's lactate solution at approximately 200 to 250 ml/hr of operative procedure.

Arrhythmias

Alteration from normal sinus rhythm may occur during the operative procedure [5-97]. Minor arrhythmias may occur in most patients, and have been reported in up to 84 per cent in some series. In the past these have often been missed when continuous electrocardiographic monitoring was not performed. The majority of patients show supraventricular arrhythmias consisting mainly of premature atrial or premature atrioventricular nodal contractions. A significant number of patients develop ventricular arrhythmias, usually premature ventricular contractions; some develop both supraventricular and ventricular arrhythmias. The greatest incidence of arrhythmias occurs during anesthesia and operative manipulation, with the highest frequency related to intubation and a somewhat lesser frequency related to extubation. Patients with a history of cardiac disease show a significantly higher percentage of arrhythmic episodes and tend to have more ventricular arrhythmias.

Therapy for Arrhythmias

It appears clear that cardiac arrhythmias are associated with anoxia, acidosis, and anesthesia. Such arrhythmias, especially premature ventricular contractions, are indicative of a potentially dangerous or even fatal outcome if immediate therapy is not undertaken. Ventricular arrhythmias may progress to fibrillation or cardiac arrest.

CHECK FOR ANESTHESIA, ANOXIA, ACIDOSIS

The adequacy of ventilation should be immediately checked by observing the movement of air and drawing an arterial blood gas. Precise check of any drugs and gases being administered to the patient should be made, and if the arrhythmia continues these drugs should be stopped and the patient ventilated with pure oxygen or room air. If difficulties in ventilation are detected either by the inability to move air easily in and out of the lungs or by alterations in the arterial gas levels, auscultation of the chest should be performed. The endotracheal tube balloon should be deflated, and immediate consideration given to replacing the endotracheal tube. It should be emphasized that it is possible for the endotracheal balloon to occlude the orifice of the endotracheal tube, for the tube to be advanced into the right mainstem bronchus with nonventilation of the left lung, and for the tube to be partially occluded by secretions, allowing some gas flow and even the passage of an endotracheal suction catheter, but not permitting adequate ventilatory exchange. If there is any question whatsoever about the adequacy of ventilation, the patient should be disconnected from all anesthesia equipment and ventilated by an Ambu bag or by mouth-to-tube ventilation. Mechanical problems do occur in anesthesia machines, gauges, valves, and in endotracheal tubes which are capable of interfering with adequate ventilation during operative procedures.

DRUG THERAPY

If complete evaluation of the patient's condition indicates that ventilation is adequate, that there is no excessive drug administration, and that anoxia or acidosis are not present as proved by blood gas determination, intravenous lidocaine or quinidine can be used. The decision as to whether to proceed with the operative procedure must be made in the individual case, depending upon the need for operation and the stage of the operative procedure at which the arrhythmia occurred.

POSTOPERATIVE CARE

Careful attention to the clinical state of the patient and proper use of monitoring, both electrical and chemical, is essential. Cardiac rate and rhythm, blood pressure, skin color and turgor, central venous pressure, urine output, chest auscultation, blood gases, and mental state remain the important parameters.

MANAGEMENT OF LOW-CARDIAC-OUTPUT SYNDROME

Normally the cardiac output varies between 2.5 and 4.5 liters/min/sq m of body surface. Studies using controlled flow while on cardiopulmonary bypass have shown that a minimum of 1.2 liters/min/sq m is required for basal metabolism, and that below this level progressive acidosis develops [5-98]. Levels of cardiac output between 1.2 and 2.0 to 2.2 liters/min/sq m may not produce progressive acidosis, but provide inadequate circulation to many vital tissues, especially the liver and kidneys [5-99]. Continuation of this low-flow state eventually leads to deterioration of vital organ systems, including the heart itself.

Volume Replacement

Treatment of the low-cardiac-output syndrome requires first that volume deficits be replaced to bring the central venous pressure at least into the high normal range. The composition of the circulating blood both in red blood cells and chemical elements must be returned to normal and acidosis corrected. Adequate oxygenation and removal of carbon dioxide must be assured by attention to proper ventilation. Oncotic pressure of the circulating plasma should be restored by judicious infusions of albumin and any hypotonicity reversed by the use of diuretics, usually ethacrynic acid or furosemide.

Digitalis

In the presence of continued low cardiac output with high normal, or high venous pressure, digitalis is the first therapeutic preparation to be used. The usual preparations are digoxin and digitoxin. Digoxin differs from digitoxin in that it exists free in the plasma and is excreted unchanged in the urine. It has a biologic half-life of approximately 31 hr. Digitoxin is metabolized in the liver and exists more than 90 per cent bound to serum protein. Only about 8 per cent is excreted unchanged in the urine. Thus the rate of metabolism of digitoxin can be effected by liver disease and by drugs that affect liver function. Since both drugs are eventually excreted chiefly by the kidney, dosages must be reduced in cases of renal failure [5-100].

DIGITALIS TOXICITY

The administration of digitalis must be monitored carefully and the patient watched for signs of digitalis toxicity. The frequency of occurrence of digitalis toxicity and its dangerous sequelae have been recognized in the last few years, especially since the advent of a radioimmunoassay for serum levels [5-101]. In one study of 931 patients, 23 per cent were definitely toxic, 6 per cent possibly digitalis-toxic. Mortality in these patients was twice that in the nontoxic patients. Toxicity was usually associated with normal doses of digitalis in patients in renal failure. In addition, the toxic patients showed a higher incidence of acute or chronic pulmonary disease, and such patients appeared to be sensitive to digitalis [5-102]. The elderly patient with advanced heart disease and especially with underlying atrial fibrillation appears to be at increased risk while receiving digitalis.

Clinical signs of digitalis toxicity were manifested by disturbances in rhythm, especially atrioventricular junctional disturbances. The most common arrhythmias were atrioventricular junctional escape rhythm, ventricular bigeminy or trigeminy, nonparoxysmal atrioventricular junctional tachycardia, ectopic ventricular beats, multifocal ventricular ectopic beats or ventricular tachycardia, and atrioventricular exit block [5-103].

INOTROPIC AGENTS

If, following digitalization, cardiac output still is inadequate, other inotropic agents should be used. The administration of potent vasoactive drugs requires careful and continuous monitoring of the arterial blood pressure. Arterial catheterization with direct pressure readings is frequently required due to the possibility of error in measuring blood pressure by the usual cuff technique [5-104]. Maintenance of an adequate perfusion pressure is important to allow blood flow to the myocardium itself, especially in patients who have significant stenoses in the coronary arteries [5-105].

Isoproterenol is a beta-inotropic and chronotropic stimulator which can increase cardiac output while decreasing total peripheral vascular resistance. Such a combination of effects appears to be valuable in increasing cardiac performance in the experimental animal [5-106] and in some patients in cardiogenic shock [5-107]. It has been shown, however, that in certain instances the use of isoproterenol may cause a worsening of myocardial metabolism [5-108].

The more potent beta-adrenergic cardiac inotropic agents—norepinephrine and epinephrine—appear to produce an increase in cardiac output without significant peripheral vasoconstriction when administered in low doses [5-109], and if excess rise in blood pressure is prevented, myocardial metabolism is improved [5-108, 5-110].

Angiotensin and metaraminol appear to be less reliable in improving cardiac output and in some cases may cause a fall in cardiac output [5-107].

Glucagon has been shown to produce an increase in cardiac output and an improvement in ventricular function in critically ill patients [5-111].

Arrhythmias

The more frequent use of electrocardiographic monitoring in the acutely ill patient has exposed the dangerous and frequently lethal nature of cardiac arrhythmias.

BRADYCARDIA

Bradycardia can be tolerated until the pulse rate falls below 40/min. If slower rates or ventricular asystole occur, treatment must be immediate. Drug therapy is limited and electrical pacing must be instituted at once [5-112].

TACHYCARDIA

Tachycardias may be tolerated up to rates of 140 to 150/min in patients with normal myocardial reserve. However, rates of 100 to 120/min may not be tolerated by patients with poor myocardial reserve.

Supraventricular Arrhythmias. The supraventricular tachyarrhythmias, atrial tachycardia, atrial flutter, and atrial fibrillation, rarely are emergency problems if ventricular rates are maintained within the normal range. Cardiac output does fall approximately 20 per cent. Such atrial arrhythmias may be serious, however, in the patient with recent myocardial infarction. Treatment usually requires digitalization and the reversal of the arrhythmia by precordial D.C. shock. Prevention of further atrial arrhythmias may be accomplished by the administration of propranalol or quinidine.

Junctional Arrhythmias. Junctional tachycardias usually result from an excess of digitalis. Withdrawal of this drug is indicated with correction of the electrolyte imbalance, usually hypokalemia. Potassium chloride may be infused at a rate of 0.25 mEq to 0.5 mEq/min for short periods, and at rates of 10 mEq/hr for several hours with frequent measurement of serum potassium levels.

Ventricular Arrhythmias. Ventricular tachycardia and fibrillation are serious arrhythmias and can cause sudden death. The appearance of ventricular premature contractions is the indication for an immediate check of the depth of anesthesia, and for the presence of anoxia or acidosis. Rapid correction of any of these commonly present factors must be done.

Control of Arrhythmias

DRUGS

Control of ventricular arrhythmias may be obtained by an immediate intravenous bolus of 100 mg of lidocaine. This may be followed by an intravenous drip of 2 to 4 mg/min up to a maximum dose of 750 mg. For long-term control, quinidine, pronestyl, or dilantin may be used. The effectiveness of the latter two drugs may be improved by simultaneous administration of propranalol.

PACING AND DEFIBRILLATION

Electrical pacing of the heart may, in addition, be required. If ventricular fibrillation occurs, cardiac massage must be instituted and ventilation carried out to provide adequate oxygenation and prevent respiratory acidosis. Electric defibrillation should be used. If the heart proves resistant to defibrillation, administration of intracardiac epinephrine and systemic intravenous sodium bicarbonate may improve the chances of resuscitation. Blood gases should be drawn to monitor such therapy [5-113].

Use of Steroids

Corticosteroids have been suggested as an aid in the support of the circulation in shock states. It is clear that in the usual shock state adrenal cortical failure is not present, and secretion of corticosteroids is markedly elevated while catabolism is decreased. However, it has also been shown that pharmacologic concentrations of glucocorticoids administered prior to shock increase survival in a variety of shock conditions. The mechanism of this glucocorticoid protective action appears to be related to lysosomal membrane stabilization. Such stabilization would, theoretically, tend to prevent the release of myocardial depressant factor from the anoxic liver [5-114]. The precise value of corticosteroid therapy in the treatment of cardiogenic shock is not yet known.

REFERENCES

5-1. Stenger, R. J., and Spiro, D.: Structure of the cardiac muscle cell. Am. J. Med. 30:653, 1961.

5-2. Fawcett, D. W.: The sarcoplasmic reticulum of skeletal and cardiac muscle. Circulation 24:336, 1961.

5-3. Woodbury, J. W.: Cellular electrophysiology of the heart, in Hamilton, W. F., and Dow, P. (eds.), Handbook of physiology, Sec. 2: Circulation. Vol. 1. Washington, D.C., American Physiological Society, 1962, pp. 237–286.

5-4. Spiro, D., and Sonnenblick, E. H.: Comparison of the ultrastructural basis of the contractile process in heart and skeletal muscle. Circ. Res. (Suppl.) 2:II-14, 1964.

5-5. Page, S. G., and Huxley, H. E.: Filament lengths in striated muscle. J. Cell Biol. 19:369, 1963.

5-6. Huxley, A. F., and Niedergerke, R.: Structural changes in muscle during contraction. Interference microscopy of living muscle fibres. Nature 173:971, 1954.

5-7. Huxley, H. E.: Muscle Cells. In J. Brachet and A. E .Mirsky (eds.), The Cell; Biochemistry, Physiology, and Morphology. Vol. 4, Specialized Cells, Part 1. New York, Academic Press, 1960, pp. 365–481.

5-8. Fanburg, B., Finkel, R. M., and Martonosi, A.: The role of calcium in the mechanism of relaxation of cardiac muscle. J. Biol. Chem. 239:2298, 1964.

5-9. Costantin, L. L., Franzini-Armstrong, C., and Podolsky, R. J.: Localization of calcium-accumulating structures in striated muscle fibers. Science 147:158, 1965.

5-10. Frank, O.: Zur Dynamik des Herzmuskels. Zeitschr. F. Biol. 32: 370, 1895.

5-11. Starling, E. H.: The Lineacre lecture on the law of the heart. Given at Cambridge, 1915. London, Longmans, 1918.

5-12. Sonnenblick, E. H., Spiro, D., and Cottrell, T. S.: Fine structural changes in heart muscle in relation to the length-tension curve. Proc. Natl. Acad. Sci. 49:193, 1963.

5-13. Gordon, A. M., Huxley, A. F., and Julian, F. J.: The variation in isometric tension with sarcomere length in vertebrate muscle fibres. J. Physiol. 184:170, 1966.

5-14. Braunwald, E., Ross, J., Jr., and Sonnenblick, E. H.: Mechanisms of contraction of the normal and failing heart. New Engl. J. Med. 277:794, 1967.

5-15. Sonnenblick, E. H.: Force-velocity relations in mammalian heart muscle. Am. J. Physiol. 202:931, 1962.

5-16. Abbott, B. C., and Mommaerts, W. F. H. M.: A study of inotropic mechanisms in the papillary muscle preparation. J. Gen. Physiol. 42:533, 1959.

5-17. Sonnenblick, E. H.: Implications of muscle mechanics in the heart. Fed. Proc. 21:975, 1962.

5-18. Sonnenblick, E. H., Braunwald, E., and Morrow, A. G.: The contractile properties of human heart muscle: Studies on myocardial mechanics of surgically excised papillary muscles. J. Clin. Invest. 44:966, 1965.

5-19. Glick, G., Sonnenblick, E. H., and Braunwald, E.: Myocardial force-velocity relations studied in intact unanesthetized man. J. Clin. Invest. 44:978, 1965.

5-20. Sarnoff, S. J., and Mitchell, J. H.: Control of function of heart.

In W. F. Hamilton and P. Dow (eds.) Handbook of Physiology; Section 2, Circulation, Vol. I. Washington, D.C., Am. Physiol. Soc., 1962, Chapt. 15, pp. 489–532.

5-21. Patterson, S. W., and Starling, E. H.: On the mechanical factors which determine the output of the ventricles. J. Physiol. 48:357, 1914.

5-22. von Anrep, G.: On the part played by the suprarenals in the normal vascular reactions of the body. J. Physiol. 45:307, 1912.

5-23. DeGeest, H., Levy, M. N., Zieske, H., and Lipman, R. I.: Depression of ventricular contractility by stimulation of the vagus nerves. Circ. Res. 17:222, 1965.

5-24. Cooper, T., Gilbert, J. W., Jr., Bloodwell, R. D., and Crout, J. R.: Chronic extrinsic cardiac denervation by regional neural ablation: Description of the operation, verification of the denervation, and its effects on myocardial catecholamines. Circ. Res. 9:275, 1961.

5-25. Donald, D. E., Milburn, S. E., and Shepherd, J. T.: Effect of cardiac denervation on the maximal capacity for exercise in the racing greyhound. J. Appl. Physiol. 19:849, 1964.

5-26. Hoffman, B. F., Bindler, E., and Suckling, E. E.: Postextrasystolic potentiation of contraction in cardiac muscle. Am. J. Physiol. 185:95, 1956.

5-27. Ross, J., Jr., Sonnenblick, E. H., Kaiser, G. A., Frommer, P. L., and Braunwald, E.: Electroaugmentation of ventricular performance and oxygen consumption by repetitive application of paired electrical stimuli. Circ. Res. 16:332, 1965.

5-28. Monroe, R. G., and French, G. N.: Left ventricular pressure-volume relationships and myocardial oxygen consumption in the isolated heart. Circ. Res. 9:362, 1961.

5-29. Krasnow, N., Rolett, E. L., Yurchak, P. M., Hood, W. B., Jr., and Gorlin, R.: Isoproterenol and cardiovascular performance. Am. J. Med. 37:514, 1964.

5-30. Sonnenblick, E. H., Ross, J., Jr., Covell, J. W., Kaiser, G., and Braunwald, E.: Velocity of contraction: A major determinant of myocardial oxygen consumption. (Abstr.) J. Clin. Invest. 44:1099, 1965.

5-31. Bing, R. J.: Cardiac metabolism. Physiol. Rev. 45:171, 1965.

5-32. Scheuer, J., and Brachfeld, N.: Coronary insufficiency: Relations between hemodynamic, electrical, and biochemical parameters. Circ. Res. 18:178, 1966.

5-33. Guyton, A. C.: Circulatory Physiology. Cardiac Output and Its Regulation. Philadelphia, Saunders, 1963, p. 314.

5-34. Crawford, D. G., Fairchild, H. M., and Guyton, A. C.: Oxygen lack as a possible cause of reactive hyperemia. Am. J. Physiol. 197:613, 1959.

5-35. Barcroft, H., Dornhorst, A. C., McClatchey, H. M., and Tanner, I. M.: On the blood flow through rhythmically contracting muscle before and during release of sympathetic vasoconstrictor tone. J. Physiol. 117:391, 1952.

5-36. Gorlin, R., and Lewis, B. M.: Circulatory adjustments to hypoxia in dogs. J. Appl. Physiol. 7:180, 1954.

5-37. Richardson, T. Q., and Guyton, A. C.: Effects of polycythemia and anemia on cardiac output and other circulatory factors. Am. J. Physiol. 197:1167, 1959.

5-38. Huckabee, W. E.: Circulatory response to cytochrome oxidase inhibition in vivo. (Abstr.) Fed. Proc. 19:119, 1960.

5-39. Guyton, A. C.: Circulatory Physiology. Cardiac output and its regulation. Philadelphia, Saunders, 1963, p. 313.

5-40. Sonnenblick, E. H., Braunwald, E., Williams, J. F., Jr., and Glick, G.: Effects of exercise on myocardial force-velocity relations in intact unanesthetized man: Relative roles of changes in heart rate, sympathetic activity, and ventricular dimensions. J. Clin. Invest. 44:2051, 1965.

5-41. Albrecht, M., and Clowes, G. H. A., Jr.: The increase of circulatory requirements in the presence of inflammation. Surgery 56:158, 1964.

5-42. Gump, F. E., Price, J. B., Jr., and Kinney, J. M.: Blood flow and oxygen consumption in patients with severe burns. Surg. Gynec. Obst. 130:23, 1970.

5-43. Shoemaker, W. C., Mohr, P. A., Printen, K. J., Brown, R. S., Amato, J. J., Carey, J. S., Youssef, S., Reinhard, J. M., Kim, S. I., and Kark, A. E.: Use of sequential physiologic measurements for evaluation and therapy of uncomplicated septic shock. Surg. Gynec. Obst. 131:245, 1970.

5-44. MacLean, L. D., Mulligan, W. G., McLean, A. P. H., and Duff, J. H.: Patterns of septic shock in man—a detailed study of 56 patients. Ann. Surg. 166:543, 1966.

5-45. DelGuercio, L. R. M., Commaraswamy, R. P., Feins, N. R., Wollman, S. B., and State, D.: Pulmonary arteriovenous admixture and the hyperdynamic cardiovascular state in surgery for portal hypertension. Surgery 56:57, 1964.

5-46. Rushmer, R. F.: Cardiovascular Dynamics. Philadelphia, Saunders, 1961, p. 196.

5-47. Wang, Y., Marshall, R. J., and Shepherd, J. T.: The effect of changes in posture and of graded exercise on stroke volume in man. J. Clin. Invest. 39:1051, 1960.

5-48. Miller, D. E., Gleason, W. L., Whalen, R. E., Morris, J. J., Jr., and McIntosh, H. D.: Effect of ventricular rate on the cardiac output in the dog with chronic heart block. Circ. Res. 10:658, 1962.

5-49. Anzola, J., and Rushmer, R. F.: Cardiac responses to sympathetic stimulation. Circ. Res. 4:302, 1956.

5-50. Spann, J. F., Jr., Buccino, R. A., Sonnenblick, E. H., and Braunwald, E.: Contractile state of the myocardium in ventricular hypertrophy and heart failure. (Abstr.) Circulation 34:III-222, 1966.

5-51. Gault, J. H., Ross, J., Jr., Sonnenblick, E. H., and Braunwald, E.: Characterization of myocardial contractility in patients with and without cardiac dysfunction by the instantaneous tension-velocity relation. (Abstr.) Circulation 34:III-108, 1966.

5-52. Chidsey, C. A., Sonnenblick, E. H., Morrow, A. G., and Braunwald, E.: Norepinephrine stores and contractile force of papillary muscle from the failing human heart. Circulation 33:43, 1966.

5-53. Spann, J. F., Jr., Chidsey, C. A., and Braunwald, E.: Reduction of cardiac stores of norepinephrine in experimental heart failure. Science 145:1439, 1964.

5-54. Shaffer, A. B., and Katz, L. N.: Hemodynamic alterations in congestive heart failure. New Engl. J. Med. 276:853, 1967.

5-55. Folse, R., and Braunwald, E.: Determination of fraction of left ventricular volume ejected per beat and of ventricular end-diastolic and residual volumes. Circulation 25:674, 1962.

5-56. Levine, H. J., Neill, W. A., Wagman, R. J., Krasnow, N., and Gorlin, R.: The effect of exercise on mean left ventricular ejection rate in man. J. Clin. Invest. 41:1050, 1962.

5-57. Harrison, T. R., Calhoun, J. A., Cullen, G. E., Wilkins, W. E., and Pilcher, C.: Studies in congestive heart failure. XV. Reflex versus chemical factors in the production of rapid breathing. J. Clin. Invest. 11:133, 1932.

5-58. Page, D. L., Caulfield, J. B., Kastor, J. A., DeSanctis, R. W., and Sanders, C. A.: Myocardial changes associated with cardiogenic shock. New Engl. J. Med. 285:133, 1971.

5-59. Shoemaker, W. C.: Sequential hemodynamic patterns in various causes of shock. Surg. Gynec. Obst. 132:411, 1971.

5-60. Carey, J. S., Mohr, P. A., Brown, R. S., and Shoemaker, W. C.: Cardiovascular function in hemorrhage, trauma and sepsis: Determinants of cardiac output and cardiac work. Ann. Surg. 170:910, 1969.

5-61. Clowes, G. H. A., Jr., Sabga, G. A., Konitaxis, A., Tomin, R., Hughes, M., and Simeone, F. A.: Effects of acidosis on cardiovascular function in surgical patients. Ann. Surg. 154:524, 1961.

5-62. Goodyer, A. V. N., Goodkind, M. J., and Stanley, E. J.: The effects of abnormal concentrations of the serum electrolytes on left ventricular function in the intact animal. Am. Heart J. 67:779, 1964.

5-63. Kittle, C. F., Aoki, H., and Brown, E. B., Jr.: The role of pH and CO_2 in the distribution of blood flow. Surgery 57:139, 1965.

5-64. Andersen, M. N., and Mouritzen, C.: Effect of acute respiratory and metabolic acidosis on cardiac output and peripheral resistance. Ann. Surg. 163:161, 1966.

5-65. Thrower, W. B., Darby, T. D., and Aldinger, E. E.: Acid-base derangements and myocardial contractility. Arch. Surg. 82:56, 1961.

5-66. Smith, N. T., and Corbascio, A. N.: Myocardial resistance to metabolic acidosis. Arch. Surg. 92:892, 1966.

5-67. Brand, E. D., and Lefer, A. M.: Myocardial depressant factor in plasma from cats in irreversible post-oligemic shock. Proc. Soc. Exp. Biol. Med. 122:200, 1966.

5-68. Lundsgaard-Hansen, P.: Oxygen supply and anaerobic metabolism of the heart in experimental hemorrhagic shock. Ann. Surg. 163:10, 1966.

5-69. Williams, L. F., Jr., Goldberg, A. H., Polansky, B. J., and Byrne, J. J.: Myocardial effects of intestinal ischemia. J. Surg. Res. 9:319, 1969.

5-70. Wangensteen, S. L., Geissinger, W. T., Lovett, W. L., Glenn, T. M., and Lefer, A. M.: Relationship between splanchnic blood flow and a myocardial depressant factor in endotoxin shock. Surgery 69:410, 1971.

5-71. Wangensteen, S. L., deHoll, J. D., Kiechel, S. F., Martin, J., and Lefer, A. M.: Influence of hemodialysis on a myocardial depressant factor in hemorrhagic shock. Surgery 67:935, 1970.

5-72. Rutherford, B. D., McCann, W. D., and O'Donovan, T. P. B.: The value of monitoring pulmonary artery pressure for early detection of left ventricular failure following myocardial infarction. Circulation 43:655, 1971.

5-73. Forrester, J. S., Diamond, G., McHugh, T. J., and Swan, H. J. C.: Filling pressures in the right and left sides of the heart in acute myocardial infarction. A reappraisal of central-venous-pressure monitoring. New Engl. J. Med. 285:190, 1971.

5-74. Border, J. R.: Bedside study of the surgical patient. J. Surg. Res. 7:591, 1967.

5-75. Mauney, F. M., Jr., Ebert, P. A., and Sabiston, D. C., Jr.: Postoperative myocardial infarction: A study of predisposing factors, diagnosis, and mortality in a high risk group of surgical patients. Ann. Surg. 172:497, 1970.

5-76. Hamilton, W. F., Moore, J. W., Kinsman, J. M., and Spurling, R. G.: Studies on the circulation. IV. Further analysis of the injection method, and of changes in hemodynamics under physiological and pathological conditions. Am. J. Physiol. 99:534, 1932.

5-77.   Jacobs, R. R., Williams, B. T., and Schenk, W. G., Jr.: Cardiac
        output in hypovolemia. An evaluation of the dye dilution method
        using the electromagnetic flowmeter as a standard. Arch. Surg.
        102:199, 1971.

5-78.   Giannelli, S., Jr., Ayres, S. M., Vastola, J. W., Goldstone, R. A.,
        and Buehler, M. E.: Indicator-dilution curves obtained across
        the systemic circulation during cardiopulmonary bypass perfu-
        sion. Surgery 57:423, 1965.

5-79.   Carey, J. S., and Hughes, R. K.: Cardiac output. Clinical monitor-
        ing and management. Ann. Thorac. Surg. 7:150, 1969.

5-80.   Edwards, A. W. T., Bassingthwaighte, J. B., Stutterer, W. F., and
        Wood, E. H.: Blood level of indocyanine green in the dog dur-
        ing multiple dye curves and its effect on instrumental calibration.
        Proc. Staff Meeting Mayo Clinic. 35:745, 1960.

5-81.   Burton, A. C.: Physiology and biophysics of the circulation. Chi-
        cago, Year Book Medical Publishers, 1965.

5-82.   Hamilton, W. F.: Measurement of the cardiac output. In W. F.
        Hamilton (ed.), Handbook of Physiology, Sec. 2. Circulation,
        Vol. 1. Washington, American Physiological Society, 1962, pp.
        551–584.

5-83.   Conn, H. L., Jr.: Use of external counting technics in studies of
        the circulation. Circ. Res. 10:505, 1962.

5-84.   Kinsman, J. M., Moore, J. W., and Hamilton, W. F.: Studies on
        the circulation. 1. Injection method: physical and mathematical
        considerations. Am. J. Physiol. 89:322, 1939.

5-85.   Warner, H. R., Gardner, R. M., and Toronto, A. F.: Computer-
        based monitoring of cardiovascular functions in postoperative
        patients. Circulation (suppl. 2) 67–68: II-74, 1968.

5-86.   Warner, H. R.: The role of computers in medical research. JAMA,
        196:944, 1966.

5-87.   Kouchoukos, N. T., Sheppard, L. C., McDonald, D. A., and
        Kirklin, J. W.: Estimation of stroke volume from the central
        arterial pressure contour in postoperative patients. Surg. Forum
        20:180, 1969.

5-88.   Kubicek, W. G., Karegis, J. N., Patterson, R. P., Witsoe, D. A.,
        and Mattson, R. H.: Development and evaluation of an imped-
        ance cardiac output system. Aerospace Med. 37:1208, 1966.

5-89.   Harley, A., and Greenfield, J. C., Jr.: Determination of cardiac
        output in man by means of impedance plethysmography. Aero-
        space Med. 39:248, 1968.

5-90.   Siegel, J. H., Fabian, M., Lankau, C., Levine, M., Cole, A., and
        Nahmad, M.: Clinical and experimental use of thoracic im-
        pedance plethysmography in quantifying myocardial contractility.
        Surgery 67:907, 1970.

5-91.   Gudwin, A. L., Goldstein, C. R., Cohn, J. D., Del Guercio, L. R.:
        Estimation of ventricular mixing volume for prediction of opera-
        tive mortality in the elderly. Ann. Surg. 168:183, 1968.
5-92.   Siegel, J. H., and Williams, J. B.: A Computer-based index for the
        prediction of operative survival in patients with cirrhosis and
        portal hypertension. Ann. Surg. 169:191, 1969.
5-93.   Spodick, D. H., Dorr, C. A., and Calabrese, B.: Detection of car-
        diac abnormality by clinical measurement of left ventricular
        ejection time: a prospective study of 200 unselected patients.
        JAMA 209:239, 1969.
5-94.   Mazzia, V. D. B., Ellis, C. H., Siegel, H., and Hershey, S. G.: The
        Electrocardiograph as a monitor of cardiac function in the
        operating room. JAMA 198:103, 1966.
5-95.   Folkow, B., Gelin, L. E., Lindell, S. E., Stenberg, K., and
        Thoren, O.: Cardiovascular reaction during abdominal surgery.
        Ann. Surg. 156:905, 1962.
5-96.   Bertrand, C. A., Steiner, N. V., Jameson, A. G., and Lopez, M.:
        Disturbances of cardiac rhythm during anesthesia and surgery.
        JAMA 216:1615, 1971.
5-97.   Kuner, J., Enesou, V., Utsu, F., Boszormenyi, E., Bernstein, H., and
        Corday, E.: Cardiac arrhythmias during anesthesia. Dis. Chest
        52:580, 1976.
5-98.   Clowes, G. H. A., Jr.: Extracorporeal maintenance of circulation
        and respiration. Physiol. Rev. 40:826, 1960.
5-99.   Mundth, E. D., Keller, A. R., and Austen, W. G.: Progressive
        hepatic and renal failure associated with low cardiac output
        following open-heart surgery. J. Thorac. Cardiovasc. Surg. 53:
        275, 1967.
5-100. DeGraff, A. C.: A new look at an old standby. Cardiovasc. Rev.,
        Medical World News, 1971, pg. 71.
5-101. Beller, G. A., Smith, T. W., Abelmann, W. H., Haber, E., and
        Hood, W. B., Jr.: Digitalis intoxication: a prospective clinical
        study with serum level correlations. New Engl. J. Med. 284:989,
        1971.
5-102. Baum, G. L., Dick, M. M., Blum, A., Kaupe, A., and Carballo, J.:
        Factors involved in digitalis sensitivity in chronic pulmonary
        insufficiency. Am. Heart J. 57:460, 1959.
5-103. Smith, T. H., and Haber, E.: Digoxin intoxication: the relationship
        of clinical presentation to serum digoxin concentration. J. Clin.
        Invest. 49:2377, 1970.
5-104. Cohn, J. N., and Luria M. H.: Studies in clinical shock and hypo-
        tension: The value of bedside hemodynamic observations. JAMA
        190:113, 1964.
5-105. Gunnar, R. M., Loeb, H. S., Pietras, R. J., and Tobin, J. R.: In-

effectiveness of isoproterenol in shock due to acute myocardial infarction. JAMA 202:1124, 1967.

5-106.   Bloch, J. H., Pierce, C. H., Manax, W. G., and Lillehei, R. C.: Treatment of experimental cardiogenic shock. Surgery 58:197, 1965.

5-107.   Smith, H. J., Oriol, A., Morch, J., and McGregor, M.: Hemodynamic studies in cardiogenic shock: treatment with isoproterenol and metaraminol. Circulation 35:1084, 1967.

5-108.   Mueller, H., Ayres, S. M., Gregory, J. J., Giannelli, S., Jr., and Grace, W. J.: Hemodynamics, coronary blood flow, and myocardial metabolism in coronary shock: response to L-norepinephrine and isoproterenol. J. Clin. Invest. 49:1885, 1970.

5-109.   Clauss, R. H., and Ray, J. F., III.: Pharmacologic assistance to the failing circulation. Surg. Gynec. Obst., 126:611, 1968.

5-110.   Cohn, J. N., and Luria, M. H.: Studies in clinical shock and hypotension. II. Hemodynamic effects of norepinephrine and angiotensin. J. Clin. Invest. 44:1494, 1965.

5-111.   Siegel, J. H., Levine, M. J., McConn, R., and Del Guercio, L. R. M.: The effect of glucagon infusion on cardiovascular function in the critically ill. Surg. Gynec. Obst. 131:505, 1970.

5-112.   Escher, D. J. W., and Furman, S.: Emergency treatment of cardiac arrhythmias: emphasis on use of electrical pacing. JAMA 214:2028, 1970.

5-113.   Redding, J. S., and Pearson, J. W.: Resuscitation from ventricular fibrillation: drug therapy. JAMA 203:93, 1968.

5-114.   Lefer, A. M., and Verrier, R. L.: Role of corticosteroids in the treatment of circulatory collapse states. Clin. Pharmacol. Ther. 11:630, 1970.

6

BODY FLUIDS

BODY WATER

Most of the bulk of the human body is water. The average 70-kg man has a body surface area of 1.73 sq m, and a total body water of approximately 43 liters (60 to 65 per cent of body weight). Of this total body fluid, extracellular water makes up approximately 12 liters (16 to 18 per cent of body weight), and intracellular water 31 liters (approximately 45 per cent of body weight). In this average individual, the blood volume measures 5 liters of which 2.8 are plasma and 2.2 red cell mass [6-1]. The 16 kg of total body fat-free solids are dispersed in the intra- and extracellular water. The remainder of the body, 11 kg, is made up of fat.

Fluid Water

For the most part, body water exists as a structural composite, for very little can be found in the liquid form. The liquid phases of total body water are the plasma and the lymph, plus those small amounts contained in specialized organ spaces, such as visceral fluids and cerebrospinal fluid. Plasma volume normally occupies 5 per cent of the body weight or 7.5 per cent of the total body water. The actual volume of liquid lymph has never been precisely determined. A calculation can be made on the basis of lymph albumin. Albumin in the extravascular space is contained in the lymph, and by dilutional studies has been found to equal the total intravascular circulating albumin

[6-2, 6-3]. Lymph albumin concentration is approximately 50 to 60 per cent of that in the plasma. It can, therefore, be estimated that the fluid lymph volume is approximately two times the plasma volume. Some estimates have placed lymph volume at one to one and one-half times the total blood volume [6-4]. Thus the circulating liquid lymph volume makes up 12 to 14 per cent of the total body water. The total plasma and lymph in liquid form are 20 per cent of the total body water, while 80 per cent of the body water is intracellular or in the connective tissue in a structured form.

Structured Water

Water, even in the liquid form, exists partially as a monomer and partially as a polymer, with a hexagonal structure enclosing a positive ion. These forms are constantly interchanging at a very rapid rate with a molecular lifetime of 10^{-11} sec [6-5]. Water within cells and within connective tissue is influenced by the polyanionic macromolecules of protein polysaccharides, and is held to these large molecules by electrical forces. Studies of nuclear magnetic resonance have indicated alteration in the freedom of movement of hydrogen ions under these circumstances, leading to the concept of a structured water shell surrounding the macromolecule [6-6]. Ling has shown that there are four layers of water molecules around a polar protein. Within the cell the protein chain-to-chain distance (17 Å) is such that most of cell water is polarized and held in this semifixed state [6-7].

The water content of connective-tissue ground substance is also held in layered complexes around protein polysaccharide molecules. The long-chain protein polysaccharides interlace the connective tissue ground substance to form a gel. This gel apparently exists in a state intermediate between a liquid and a solid [6-8]. The transport of solute and water through the gel is affected by the degree of stabilization of the protein-water system [6-9]. Water diffusion increases with increasing disorder of the organizing structure. The speed of diffusion also changes with changes in temperature and with changes in concentration of certain ions including hydrogen ion [6-8].

Alterations in transcapillary exchange may also be due to changes in the physical state of the ground substance [6-10]. Changes in capillary permeability due to the injection of endotoxin [6-11] and papain [6-12] may be examples of the effect of change in ground substance on capillary permeability.

BLOOD

Rheology

Normal transport of substances to and from body-tissue cells occurs by movement of whole blood within the vascular system. The composition of blood affects the characteristics of flow. The viscosity of whole blood depends primarily upon the hematocrit [6-13, 6-14]. Fibrinogen and other proteins within the plasma contribute only a small amount to total whole-blood viscosity. Platelet concentration appears to have no effect [6-15].

SHEAR EFFECTS

The actual flow rate of blood depends, in addition, on the degree of shear, with viscosity elevated at low rates of shear, decreasing as the shear rate is increased. Shear rates are proportional to the velocity of flow and inversely proportional to the radius of the vessel. Aortic blood flow with a velocity of 35 cm/sec and a radius of 1.3 cm would demonstrate quite a different shear than an end-arteriole where the flow velocity is 0.11 mm/sec and the radius 50 μ [6-16]. A decreasing vessel size should lead to an increasing shear rate and a decreasing blood viscosity. Thus, in the normal vascular system the viscosity of the blood may alter significantly in various parts of the system [6-17].

HEMATOCRIT EFFECTS

The effects of variation in hematocrit on venous return to the heart were studied by Guyton and Richardson who showed that venous return increased at a standard pressure when the hematocrit was low and decreased with elevation above normal. However, the minute flow of red blood cells to the tissues was maximal at a hematocrit of 40. Increase in cardiac output in animals with low hematocrits could not compensate for the decrease in red cell flow [6-18].

Alterations in whole-blood viscosity have been shown to occur after hemorrhage, trauma, surgical operation, and myocardial infarction [6-19, 6-20, 6-21]. Patients in postoperative shock showed significantly increased viscosity, especially at low shear rates [6-22]. This would suggest that the optimum hematocrit might be somewhat less than 40 per cent in the postoperative patient. Total peripheral resistance has been shown to be influenced both by whole blood viscosity and by the adequacy of blood volume [6-23]. However, peak oxygen delivery per minute occurs within the normal hematocrit range, irrespective of blood volume changes.

OXYGEN DELIVERY BY RED BLOOD CELLS

Oxygen delivery to the cell depends not only on the minute delivery of red cells to the tissue bed and the concentration of hemoglobin within the red cell, but also upon the interaction of hemoglobin with organic phosphates within the cell. Seventy to eighty per cent of these phosphates are present as 2,3-diphosphoglycerate (2,3-DPG)[6-24]. Synthesis of 2,3-DPG depends on the availability of adequate amounts of inorganic phosphate [6-25]. With increase in 2,3-DPG content, the position of the oxyhemoglobin dissociation curve is shifted to the right, producing a decreased affinity of hemoglobin for oxygen and increased release of oxygen to the tissues. A fall in 2,3-DPG levels produces a shift to the left with increased hemoglobin oxygen affinity and a decrease in release of oxygen to the tissues. Increase in 2,3-DPG levels has been found in situations which produce either an increased peripheral oxygen demand or a relative oxygen lack, as in patients with chronic lung disease, cyanotic heart disease, decreased red cell mass, thyrotoxicosis, and liver disease [6-26, 6-27, 6-28]. Increase also appears to occur after administration of steroids, and following elevation of pH [6-29]. A decrease in the 2,3-DPG levels was found in patients suffering from septic shock [6-24] and was lowest in those patients who did not survive. With improvement in the shock state, 2,3-DPG levels rose, sometimes above normal. Low levels of 2,3-DPG have also been found in patients with deficiencies in growth hormone and thyroxin [6-30].

Blood stored in ACD solution has been shown to have an increased oxygen affinity with a shift of the dissociation curve to the left and a parallel fall in 2,3-DPG levels [6-31]. The fall in 2,3-DPG levels in stored blood occurs progressively, and approximately 70 per cent is lost in the first three days. Although the transfused red cell can regain normal 2,3-DPG levels within 24 hours after transfusion, the metabolic defect imposed by the transfusion of large amounts of stored blood may be considerable, especially in the traumatized or septic patient.

BLOOD VOLUME REPLACEMENT

The blood volume for each individual is stabilized at a level reflecting a balance of cardiac output, total vascular resistance, and a normal distribution of body fluids. Acute disturbance of the blood volume by moderate to severe hemorrhage causes immediate hemodynamic compensation, and initiates a complex response to effect refilling of the intravascular space [6-32]. Replacement of red cell mass is a relatively slow process, depending upon cell multiplication. Replacement of plasma volume in amounts sufficient to bring total blood volume to normal occurs rapidly. Plasma refill rates as high as 90 to 120 ml/hr have been measured in the early stages after hemorrhage [6-32]. Basic to the replenishment of plasma volume is the inflow of protein from extravascular sites [6-33, 6-34] This large protein influx appears to come from existing protein residing in the extravascular pool rather than from the creation of new protein [6-35]. Transport of such protein occurs across vascular beds following a decrease in the central venous pressure and increase in catecholamine activity and from refill via the thoracic duct [6-34].

Massive Transfusion

With severe protracted hemorrhage, blood transfusion, often massive, is needed for survival. The rapidity of resuscitation with blood appears to be important in achieving this goal [6-36].

BLOOD WARMING

When large amounts of blood are required in a relatively short time, the blood should be warmed. The rapid administration of large amounts of cold blood has caused cardiac arrest and systemic hypothermia [6-37].

ACIDOSIS

The administration of large amounts (greater than 15 to 20 units) of blood stored in ACD solution has the potential of producing acidosis, since blood over 14 days old has a pH of 6.5 to 6.9 [6-38]. It has been suggested that 44.6 mEq of sodium bicarbonate (1 ampoule) be administered for every five units of bank blood to counteract this acidosis [6-39]. This formula can lead to the overadministration of sodium bicarbonate, however, and such base administration should be titrated by the blood-gas levels [6-40]. It may be that more prompt and adequate resuscitation corrects metabolic acidosis by the restoring of perfusion, thus obviating the need for administered sodium bicarbonate.

CITRATE INTOXICATION

The possibility of the production of citrate intoxication due to the administration of the ACD anticoagulant solution has been studied and apparently is not a significant factor unless large amounts of blood are administered ultrarapidly (one unit every three to four minutes). Under these rare circumstances, cardiac output may fall due to depression of ventricular contractile force, an alteration which may be corrected by the administration of calcium [6-44].

CALCIUM ADMINISTRATION

The possible dangers of calcium administration in producing ventricular irritability have been reported by Howland et al [6-42], and calcium salts are probably not needed in the ordinary blood replacement situation.

Hemorrhage During Massive Transfusion

THROMBOCYTOPENIA AND THROMBASTHENIA

A hemorrhagic state may occur following the infusion of moderate to large amounts of bank blood due to the fact that blood platelets stored in ACD solution rapidly disintegrate. The platelet count in such blood falls to 30 per cent of the initial value within 24 hr and those platelets remaining are questionably effective. Bleeding occurring in the course of multiple transfusions is thus most often due to thrombocytopenia and an immediate platelet count should be obtained [6-43]. Platelets become critical at levels below 50,000/cu ml, and may be implicated in surgical bleeding at any level under 100,000, especially if qualitative changes have taken place due to storage [6-44].

If thrombocytopenia or thrombasthenia is suspected, the treatment is the administration of 6 to 8 units of platelet concentrate. These are fresh platelets in high concentration. The use of platelet concentrate is important in order to raise the concentration of platelets in the circulating blood. The administration of fresh whole blood will not accomplish this result.

LOSS OF LABILE CLOTTING FACTORS

The more labile factors of the blood coagulation system may decrease with storage in ACD medium. Factor V is significantly decreased within 24 to 48 hr. Factor VIII is somewhat decreased with longer storage. Occasionally decreases in these factors may be responsible for abnormal bleeding, but this is rare. The use of fresh frozen plasma will restore all of these labile factors, and it is more readily available than is fresh whole blood.

Washed Red Blood Cell Transfusion

Consideration should be given to the administration of packed red blood cells when increased red cell mass is required. The use of such suspended cells removes the possibility of the development of leukocyte isoantibodies and platelet antibodies, and prevents the development of antibodies against gamma globulin [6-45]. The high plasma potassium levels (up to 25 mEq/liter) of stored blood are avoided, and the incidence of serum hepatitis carried in the plasma is decreased. It has been estimated that approximately 80 per cent of the transfusion needs of patients could be supplied by packed red cells with a dcrease in the complications caused by administering plasma, platelets, and leukocytes [6-46].

Frozen Blood

The development of a practical method for freezing red blood cells has made possible the long-term storage of blood [6-47]. This has eminent practicality from the point of view of storage and transportation, and can be used to stockpile rare forms of blood or to allow the use of autotransfusion. The red cells are administered as suspended washed red blood cells. Problems with this method are the cumbersome freezing and washing techniques and the presence of moderate amounts of free hemoglobin. In the posttransfusion plasma, free hemoglobin levels have risen 3 to 4 mg/100 ml/unit transfused [6-48].

Cadaver Blood

Cadaver blood has been used to provide transfusion in the Soviet Union for many years. Four to six units of blood may be drawn from an adult cadaver. The donor must have died a sudden death without lacerations, abrasions, infections, or cancer, and the blood must be drawn within six hours of death under sterile conditions. Large numbers of these transfusions have been used with very low complication rates

[6-49]. In the United States a major deterent to the use of cadaver blood seems to be the procurement of sufficient numbers of cadavers, as a result of sudden death without lacerations, abrasions, or infections [6-50].

Autotransfusion

A patient may be transfused with his own blood under two circumstances. Venesection may be done five to ten days prior to an elective surgical procedure and as much as two units withdrawn sequentially. This use of autotransfusion during subsequent operation has proved practical [6-51, 6-52]. Immediate autotransfusion may also be used under emergency situations if the blood has been lost into a body cavity and is not contaminated [6-53].

Blood Substitutes

Substitutes for homologous blood have been sought for several reasons. The advantages of a satisfactory blood substitute would be ready procurement and availability, and ease of administration without specific cross-matching techniques. In addition, certain adverse effects of whole homologous blood might be avoided. Investigation into blood substitutes has been divided into two areas—first, substitutes for the oxygen carrying portion of whole blood, the red cell, and second, substitutes for plasma.

OXYGEN-CARRYING SUBSTANCES
Oxygen transport to the tissues occurs primarily within red blood cells by the formation of oxyhemoglobin. Oxygen dissolved in plasma supplies only a small portion of tissue needs. In the normal individual red blood cells survive for approximately 90 days [6-54]. Cells preserved in ACD solution survive approximately 30 days. Excluding major blood group incompatibilities, homologous red cells appear to function adequately after transfusion with an average life span of approximately 14 days. The use of washed red cells can provide adequate oxygen-carrying capacity and such cells can be maintained in the frozen state for long periods of time [6-55].

Other approaches to oxygen transport have been sough, namely the use of stroma-free hemoglobin solution [6-56] and certain chemical compounds [6-57]. For the present, however, red blood cells appear to be the only practical vehicle for oxygen transport within the vascular system.

PLASMA SUBSTITUTES

Homologous plasma has certain adverse effects when transfused. Hepatitis virus may be transferred in the plasma; completely satisfactory means for detection or destruction of this virus have not yet been perfected. Transfusion of white blood cells contained in the plasma may cause the development of white-cell antibodies. Immunologic reactions may occur to certain proteins in the plasma with alteration in pulmonary vascular dynamics [6-58] or with leakage of administered plasma from the vascular space [6-59]. Certain physical changes may occur in stored plasma leading to precipitation of platelet-fibrin masses which may be damaging to the pulmonary capillary bed [6-60].

Plasma subsitutes may be used to replace limited losses of whole blood in acute hemorrhage. Loss of whole blood by hemorrhage can be replaced by Ringer's lactate solution in amounts three or four times the volume of blood lost, providing the blood loss is moderate and the hematocrit level is not allowed to fall below 28 to 30 per cent [6-61]. Serum protein levels appear to be well maintained in spite of the administration of fairly large amounts of nonprotein containing solution [6-62]. Studies of resuscitation from hemorrhagic shock comparing the use of blood, colloid, and saline show better restoration of cardiac output and flow when blood is used compared to saline alone. However, the combination of blood plus Ringer's lactate solution is preferable, perhaps because of improved flow characteristics due to hemodilution [6-63, 6-64].

Colloid solutions maintain the blood volume in a much more physiologic manner than do crystalloids [6-65]. The molecular size and the total osmolarity of the solution determines transcapillary flux of fluid. Crystalloids partition at least four to one in the extravascular space and massive infusions may produce edema in pulmonary and systemic tissues. Certain colloid plasma substitutes are hyperosmotic and cause an influx of fluid from the extravascular extracellular space [6-66]. Dextran, hydroxyethyl starch, and gelatin produce this effect. In a study by Golub et al, a mixture of colloid and crystalloid appeared to maintain a normal distribution of extracellular fluid. This combination was prepared by mixing 3 volumes of colloid (dextran or hydroxyethyl starch) with 7 volumes of lactated Ringer's solution [6-66].

Alterations in the hemostatic mechanism are produced by the infusion of certain colloid preparations. Dextran appears to decrease the tensile strength of clot, to cause prolongation of bleeding time, and an increase in spontaneous hemorrhage. Hydroxyethyl starch causes similar but less marked changes. Colloid-crystalloid mixtures cause no change in coagulation mechanisms. In their comparative study of 11 colloid plasma expander preparations, Golub et al concluded that diluted dextran, diluted hydroxyethyl starch, and a French gelatin preparation (Plasmagel-E) were the safest available plasma expanders [6-66].

There has been considerable interest in the antithrombotic effect of the dextrans, especially low-molecular-weight dextran (40,000 molecular weight). It has been suggested that the negative charge of the red cell is increased by the dextrans and that cell aggregation is therefore decreased. Most studies, however, indicate that the improved flow characteristics produced by dextran are due to decrease in blood viscosity and increase in volume due to the high oncotic pressure [6-67, 6-68, 6-69]. Flow improvement occurs only when circulating volume and cardiac output are increased [6-70].

COAGULOPATHIES IN SURGICAL PATIENTS

Several types of coagulation defects may occur in patients coming to operation.

Congenital

The congenital types of coagulopathy may be treated successfully with appropriate blood fractions. Patients with defects of Factor VIII (hemophilia) and patients with defects in Factor IX (Christmas disease) have been successfully operated upon electively [6-71]. Other less commonly encountered congenital defects include von Willebrandt's disease, congenital fibrinogen deficiency, congenital prothrombin deficiency, and deficiencies of Factors V, VII, X, XI, and XIII. Such patients have undergone operation without difficulty when appropriate fractions are administered [6-72].

Due to Trauma

Alterations in the clotting mechanism may occur following severe trauma [6-73, 6-74]. These changes vary from hypercoagulability to hypocagulability in different individuals and at different times in the same individual. There is, however, a tendency to increased fibrinolysis [6-74].

DISSEMINATED INTRAVASCULAR COAGULATION

Disseminated intravascular coagulation has been recognized as an important and often fatal complication of many serious injuries, illnesses, and infections. The possibility of such coagulation was suggested by Crowell and Reed in 1955 [6-75] and extensively studied by Hardaway [6-76, 6-77]. When carefully sought, evidence of disseminated intravascular coagulation is seen quite frequently in patients with trauma and sepsis [6-78, 6-79]. Signs of intravascular coagulation are those of hypotension, interference with peripheral circulation, cyanosis and necrosis of fingers and toes, oliguria, and the development of refractory acidosis.

Consumption Coagulopathy

The disseminated coagulation process uses up clotting factors with the production of a consumption coagulopathy and bleeding. The diagnosis of this type of coagulopathy can be made by studying the coagulation factors in the blood. It may be very difficult to differentiate it from liver disease. Factor VIII remains nearly normal in most liver disease, whereas it is decreased in consumption coagulopathy. Liver disease and coagulopathy due to multiple transfusions with washout should show more normal levels of Factors II and X since these are stable. They are, however, low in disseminated intravascular coagulation (DIC). In DIC there is a low fibrinogen clot which shows partial dissolution. Fibrinogen, Factor II, Factor V, Factor VIII, and platelets are all low. Therefore, laboratory tests show a low platelet count, increased prothrombin time, increased thrombin time, and low fibrinogen levels.

Fibrinolysis

The production of intravascular clot stimulates secondary fibrinolysis with resulting decrease in plama plasminogin, increase in the thrombin time, and an increase in the fibrin split products in the blood. Primary fibrinolysis is a rare condition and can be differentiated from the secondary type found in DIC by the presence of a normal platelet count and a normal prothrombin time in the primary form [6-80].

Treatment

Treatment depends on the precise diagnosis. Heparin has been tried with success in some cases of disseminated intravascular coagulation. It does require a degree of confidence to administer heparin to a bleeding patient, but if the situation is serious and the diagnosis quite clear, 20 to 30 mg of heparin intravenously may produce a cessation of bleeding. In addition, it may be advantageous to administer the depleted fractions and platelets.

Epsilon aminocaproic acid (EACA, Amicar) has been used to treat primary fibrinolytic states. As knowledge has increased, the absolute indications for EACA appear to be fewer. The use of this material in disseminated intravascular coagulation states may indeed be disastrous [6-81].

MICROCIRCULATION

Exchange between blood and living cells occurs across the capillary endothelial membrane. The important nutrient circulation of any tissue is, therefore, the capillary microcirculation. Capillaries are never more than 0.005 in. from any cell, and measure approximately 0.0007 in. in diameter. The total length of the capillary system of the normal adult is almost 60,000 miles, and the bulk of these capillaries is twice that of the liver [6-82].

Exchange Across the Capillary Membrane

Exchange of fluid between the blood and the extravascular space follows Starling's hypothesis. Hydrostatic pressure within the capillary exerts an outward force balanced by the inward force of osmotic pressure. The osmotic gradient is caused by large molecules in the blood, and the semipermeability of the capillary membrane. Normally outward forces predominate in the proximal capillary and inward forces in the distal capillary.

HYDROSTATIC FORCES

Change in hydrostatic pressure, change in oncotic pressure due to altered concentration of ions, or change in the permeability characteristics of the membrane, can effect fluid exchange in and out of the capillary lumen. Variations in arterial mean pressure usually do not reach the capillary bed due to the presence of precapillary arteriolar sphincters. However, elevations in mean venous pressure are transmitted to the distal capillary and may result in an increase in fluid extravasation from the capillary lumen.

Under normal conditions, the interstitial space outside the capillary wall contains fluid bound in a protein polysaccharide gel with very little mobile fluid present. What little liquid is present is rapidly drawn into the lymphatics. Normally the interstitial tissues have a negative pressure averaging −7 mm Hg [6-83]. This negative pressure is maintained by normal function of the lymphatic system and when such function ceases, tissue pressure rises with the accumulation of edema.

OSMOTIC FORCES

Plasma osmotic pressure is due primarily to the presence of albumin, although globulin and other large protein complexes contribute also. Decrease in plasma osmotic pressure due to decrease in circulating albumin allows fluid to move outward into the tissue spaces.

LYMPH

Interstitial osmotic pressure is also produced primarily by albumin, the concentration of which is regulated by the rate of lymphatic flow [6-84]. As lymph flow increases tissue osmotic pressure falls due to the removal of protein. Any interference with lymph flow allows albumin to accumulate in the interstitium, increasing the osmotic force holding fluid in the tissue. Normal lymph flow, then, is an important determinant of tissue fluid content.

LYMPH FLOW

Muscular movement appears to be an important factor in the maintenance of normal lymph flow, and decrease in flow is seen with increase in tissue pressure when anesthesia is administered [6-85]. Arterial pulsations are also an important motive force [6-86]. In the lung, normal respiratory movements are required for normal lymph flow [6-87]. The lymphatics themselves show rhythmic contracture [6-88]. Many of the factors which interfere with normal flow of lymph occur during operation and in the seriously ill patient.

PERMEABILITY FACTORS

Alterations in capillary permeability may be caused by a variety of agents. Histamine, serotonin, and bradykinin appear to cause endothelial cells to contract causing an increase in pore size. Larger molecules and accompanying water then leak into the surrounding tissues [6-89]. Hypoxia causes increased fluid movement out of the capillary lumen in peripheral and pulmonary tissue beds [6-90, 6-91, 6-92]. Endotoxin appears to effect the endothelial cells in a similar manner with increase in transcapillary transfer of large molecules [6-93]. Direct trauma and burns cause increase in capillary permeability in the local area. With severe burns of 25 to 50 per cent of the body surface area, a generalized increase in permeability may occur [6-94].

CELL-MEMBRANE TRANSPORT

The dynamics of exchange between intracellular and extracellular areas is controlled by the metabolism of the cell. Intracellular water is in osmotic equilibrium with the extracellular fluids. The differences in cation concentration with high extracellular sodium and high intracellular potassium are regulated by an energy requiring process. Cell volume as well as the specific sodium and potassium concentrations within the cell is regulated by active transport [6-95]. Conversely, energy production by the cell depends upon a normal sodium, potassium, magnesium, and calcium environment. The energy required for active transport is contained in adenosinetriphosphate (ATP), and can be released only by sodium-potassium-magnesium ATPase at the cell membrane [6-96].

Anoxia and hypothermia interfere with cell membrane transport and allow intracellular volume to increase [6-97]. The entry of glucose as energy substrate is decreased by low temperatures [6-98]. Increase in intracellular water due to a decrease in extracellular tonicity, or decrease in cell water caused by extracellular hypertonicity can cause depression of cell respiration [6-99].

ELECTROLYTE DYNAMICS

Alterations from the normal in the total amount and/or concentration of the body-fluid electrolytes cause severe disturbances in function. The need for sodium to maintain adequate extracellular fluid volume has been discussed. Potassium and magnesium are required for the functioning of most important enzyme systems [6-100]. A prime role of sodium, potassium, and magnesium is to activate ATPase to permit cell-membrane transport.

The dynamics of calcium and phosphorus is more directly related to bone metabolism, but calcium functions as an important activator of cardiac and smooth-muscle contraction. The importance of other materials found in small or trace amounts in the body is not yet known, but studies have suggested important roles for zinc [6-101, 6-102], manganese [6-103], copper [6-104], and other trace metals [6-105]. In addition, certain trace metals have been implicated in the causation of human disease [6-106].

MAINTENANCE OF BODY FLUIDS

Cells function at optimal levels under conditions of normal hydration and tonicity, and with a normal distribution of ions. Perturbations of this healthy steady state result in decrease in the efficiency of cell metabolism and thus in the efficiency of organ and organism function. Optimization of fluid volumes, distribution, tonicity, and content, is therefore important to survival of the organism when subjected to trauma and operation.

Extracellular Fluid Losses

The serious effects of extracellular dehydration have long been recognized. The first use of intravenous fluid therapy for dehydration was in 1832 [6-107, 6-108]. Extracellular dehydration has been diagnosed by changes in skin turgor and furrowing of the tongue. These signs of extracellular fluid loss were thought by Coller and Maddock to occur when 6 per cent of body weight in water had been lost [6-109]. Lapidus et al have shown that these clinical signs occur when at least 3 liters of extracellular fluid have been lost by an adult, regardless of weight [6-110].

PHYSIOLOGIC EFFECTS

Serious hemodynamic and renal decompensation can occur with loss of extracellular fluid and is proportional to that loss. Such circulatory abnormalities as decrease in the cardiac index are present even with relatively mild signs of clinical dehydration [6-111]. In the patients studied by Billig and Jordan, central venous pressure, hematocrit level, and BUN rise reflected the severity of extracellular dehydration. Cardiac index decreased proportionally as these indices indicated increasing loss.

Fluid Shifts Due to Trauma

The possibility of alteration in the distribution of body water due to acute shock and trauma has been raised by some observers. It was suggested by Shires that major deficits appeared in the extracellular fluid volume following shock and trauma [6-112]. It now appears clear that these original studies revealed primarily a change in the equilibration dynamics of certain ions, including the label ($^{35}SO_4$) used by Shires to measure extracellular fluid volume. Subsequent studies of hemorrhagic and endotoxin shock and of operation and trauma show no unexplained decrease in extracellular fluid volume [6-113, 6-114, 6-115].

An understanding of the actual fluid deficits caused by local trauma does indicate the need for extracellular fluid support in the posttrauma or postoperative patient [6-116]. The need to administer albumin to such patients has also been emphasized [6-116, 6-117, 6-118]. The administration of balanced electrolyte solution and protein in moderate amounts during protracted operative procedures, especially abdominal procedures, appears to be physiologically sound. In such patients, loss of plasma water, electrolyte, and protein into damaged tissues is sufficient to require replacement.

EVALUATION OF THE STATE OF BODY FLUIDS

History

By far the most important information concerning the body-fluid state is obtained from an adequate history and physical examination. This history should include a careful detailing of intake over the preceding 24 to 48 hours or longer. Information should be obtained concerning abnormalities of volume and tonicity, and the occurrence of any special ion lack or overload. Similar attention should be paid to the details of fluid excretion via the normal routes such as urine and sweat, or via abnormal routes. These include vomiting, loss of fluid into the intestinal tract or peritoneal cavity, loss through denuded or damaged skin, or losses from abnormal fistulae of the intestinal tract. It is possible, from a detailed history of this type, to determine with considerable accuracy the three major factors needed to define the fluid state. These are volume (is the patient over- or underhydrated?), tonicity (is the patient hyper- or hypotonic?), and problems with special ions (are there specific losses or overloads?).

Physical Examination

In the physical examination one should look for evidence to confirm the impression gained by the history. The general appearance, state of activity, and mental alertness of the patient indicate a normal or abnormal fluid state. Agitation, disorientation, and progressive coma may indicate water intoxication and hypotonicity due to water overload. Progressive decrease in mental alertness coupled with signs of tissue dehydration may indicate isotonic extracellular fluid deficit.

The physical examination should include an estimation of skin turgor. This term means the tactile estimation of fluid content and elasticity of the skin and subcutaneous areas. The skin itself may feel dry and the subcutaneous tissue may become thinned and sticky, allowing skin folds to remain elevated for an extended period of time after being picked up with the fingers. Sweat is usually absent in the axillae and groins. The mucous membranes are usually dry. However, dryness of oral mucous membranes may occur from mouth breathing in the absence of serious dehydration. Shrinking and furrowing of the tongue is a more certain sign. Softening of the eyeballs (in comparison with ones own eyeball tension) is a valuable sign but occurs late.

With progressive dehydration, the pulse may become "thready" due to depression of pulse pressure and decrease in cardiac output with peripheral vasoconstriction. Blood pressure may fall. The terminal state reveals a lack of peripheral pulses or obtainable blood pressure and extreme dryness of the tissues with coma.

Laboratory Tests

Simple laboratory tests usually suffice to confirm the condition of extracellular dehydration. The hematocrit is elevated due to loss of plasma without loss of red cell mass. However, the exact level will depend on the hematocrit which existed prior to the onset of dehydration.

Plasma chemical values may be within the normal range if isotonic loss has been occurring. A normal electrolyte pattern does not mean a normal extracellular fluid volume. If circulatory deficits have occurred, metabolic acidosis may be present with depression of the carbon dioxide content and decrease in pH. Urine will be scanty and of high specific gravity, again depending on the preexisting renal function in the particular patient. The BUN level may be elevated due to the effect of decreased cardiac output and decreased renal blood flow.

Volume Determinations

Measurements can be done by the dilutional method using radioactive labels or infused chemicals to measure extracellular fluid volumes, or red blood cell mass, or both. These are important for research information, but their use entails a sophisticated knowledge of the problems involved in using dilutional measurements in non-steady-state patients, especially those with dehydration or hemorrhage. In the normal clinical setting, such measurements are not needed except under unusual circumstances.

CORRECTION OF DEFICITS

Optimization of the fluid balance of the patient should be the aim if a successful outcome is to be attained. Volume, tonicity, and special ion problems should be brought to normal if this is at all possible. Under certain circumstances, the urgency of an operative procedure may preclude complete preoperative fluid resuscitation, and the judgment of the surgeon as to the optimum compromise between complete resuscitation and delay in operation is vital.

Assessment of Condition

Resuscitation and replacement of existing deficits depends on an accurate analysis of the fluid and electrolyte state of the patient. The history and physical examination should suffice to give information concerning volume, tonicity, and special ion problems, so that therapy may be begun. Certain guidelines should be kept in mind in initiating therapy prior to the return of any laboratory values.

VOLUME

Volume is usually decreased. Extracellular fluid deficits of 4 to 5 per cent of body weight will produce diagnosable dehydration. Extracellular fluid deficits of 10 to 12 per cent of body weight may produce death. Severe dehydration lies in the range of 6 to 8 per cent of body weight. By this calculation, a rough indication of fluid volume deficits may be made.

TONICITY

Most acute fluid losses are isotonic. This includes gastrointestinal losses by vomiting or into the intestine, peritoneal losses due to peritonitis, and transudates with loss of fluid through damaged skin or into serous cavities. Hypotonic losses may result from excessive sweating, or in a patient with an isotonic loss, who has been drinking water. Hypertonic losses occur only with direct loss of pancreatic secretions from pancreatic fistulae.

SPECIFIC ION PROBLEMS

If dehydration has persisted for some time, usually more than 24 hours, acidosis and hyponaturemia may be present. These occur due to obligatory metabolism of endogenous fat and protein with the release of free water and acid metabolites, and due to decrease in circulating plasma volume and cardiac output. In patients with chronic renal disease, the acidosis may be more severe due to the inability of the kidney to excrete hydrogen ion. In these patients fluid replacement is needed, plus support of body base by administration of sodium bicarbonate.

Metabolic alkalosis with excess loss of hydrogen ion occurs due to protracted vomiting of acid gastric contents secondary to pyloric obstruction. These patients present with a decrease in extracellular fluid and a deficit of all extracellular ions. However, the deficit of hydrogen and chloride is far in excess of other losses. Such patients require specific replacement therapy directed toward adding chloride without accompanying sodium.

Therapy

SOLUTIONS

It can be seen from the foregoing "rules of thumb" that a reasonably accurate estimate of total volume deficits can be made and that the usual resuscitative solution will be a balanced electrolyte solution for isotonic extracellular fluid support. The most commonly used solution at present is Ringer's lactate. The composition of Ringer's lactate solution approaches that of extracellular fluid with the substitution of lactate ion for bicarbonate ion. Under normal circumstances and with improvement of the patient by therapy, this lactate load poses no problem. If acidosis is present, the addition of sodium bicarbonate to the Ringer's lactate (22 mEq for each liter of Ringer's lactate) or by direct injection into the tubing, may be made. Such therapy should be monitored by serial blood gas analysis.

RATE OF ADMINISTRATION

The rate of resuscitation should be governed by the seriousness of the dehydration state, the urgency of any required surgical procedures, and the presence or absence of any chronic inadequacies of cardiovascular, pulmonary, or renal systems. In general, it should be remembered that with the institution of treatment the patient begins to improve, and therefore extremely rapid resuscitation is seldom required. In general approximately one-half of the resuscitation fluid can be given within the first three to four hours, but this rate may be cautiously increased if operation is urgent.

MONITORING OF RESPONSE

Resuscitation should be monitored by assessment of the general state of the patient by physical examination including frequent auscultation of the lungs. Measurement of the urinary output and determination of the central venous pressure should be done at regular intervals. Serial blood-gas analyses should be performed when acidosis is present. The hematocrit may be used in the absence of bleeding as a stable volume indicator to indicate the return of fluid to the intravascular space. Serum protein should be measured and albumin or plasmanate added to the resuscitative regime as indicated.

PRECAUTIONS

Several precautions are necessary. Urine volume may not increase if renal damage has been incurred during the dehydrated state. Improvement of the general condition of the patient without a rise in urine volume should alert the surgeon to this possibility, and diuresis with mannitol, ethacrynic acid, or furosemide should be started. It should be remembered that the volume of electrolyte infused is partitioned in the intra- and extravascular compartments, at a ratio of approximately one to four, and therefore, central venous pressure may not indicate accumulation of fluid in the tissues. This is especially true in conditions where capillary permeability may be increased, such as sepsis, peritonitis, pancreatitis, and burns. Interstitial edema, especially interstitial pulmonary edema, may occur unheralded by changes in central venous pressure, or by changes in sounds heard on auscultation. The only safe procedure is to exercise a high degree of caution and take interval radiographs of the chest. Such x-rays reveal the development of haziness of the lung fields prior to alterations in blood-gas values. If such interstitial pulmonary edema occurs, reduction of fluid infusion and diuresis is mandatory.

PREOPERATIVE MEASURES

A patient who is to undergo a major operative procedure, especially in the abdominal cavity, should be brought to the operating room in optimal condition as regards fluid dynamics. The usual preoperative preparation for certain intestinal procedures may produce alterations from the normal, especially dehydration. The patient may have been on an abnormal diet, perhaps low in calories. Very often he has been subjected to catharsis and enemata with resultant dehydration. Subsequently he is fasted for periods of 12 to 18 hr. Such a situation should be guarded against and appropriate preoperative therapy undertaken—usually the maintenance of normal intake for as long as possible, replacement of any abnormal fluid losses by the intravenous route, and the infusion of a preoperative fluid load of approximately one liter of Ringer's lactate solution prior to the scheduled operation.

INTRAOPERATIVE FLUID SUPPORT

During the operative procedure the patient's condition should be monitored by measurement of the central venous pressure, serial blood-gas analysis, and measurement of the urine output at 30 to 60-min intervals using an indwelling catheter. The infusion of large amounts of non-electrolyte solution should be guarded against as hypotonicity and hyponatremia are constant dangers. The anesthesiologist should be requested to record all infused volumes and to minimize the nonelectrolyte "carrier" for infused drugs. In patients undergoing major abdominal operations, especially where exposure and handling of the intestine is required, fluid is lost by evaporation and by transudation into the traumatized tissues. A fluid infusion regime of moderate proportions should be used. The administration of 200 to 300 ml of Ringer's lactate solution per hour (making a total of 2 to 3 mEq Na^+/kg for a 3 hr operation) for the adult patient undergoing major abdominal surgery will usually suffice to produce a urine output of 30 to 50 ml/hr [6-119].

Blood Replacement

A deliberate decision should be made with regard to blood replacement. If the estimated blood loss is to be 500 ml or less, one may elect to replace this with Ringer's lactate solution in 4:1 volume ratio, with added protein. Under unusual conditions, 1,000 ml of blood may be replaced in such a manner, providing that the hematocrit does not fall below the low 30's. A patient so treated, however, is in a somewhat precarious condition should massive hemorrhage then occur. If larger amounts of blood loss are unavoidable or highly probable, blood replacement should be begun to match the estimated blood loss.

Diuretics

If urine volume does not respond to the usual fluid infusion regimen, the choice lies between increasing the fluid support or the use of diuretics. This choice will depend upon the analysis of other abnormal fluid losses or transudates and upon the state of competence of the cardiovascular, pulmonary, and renal systems of the patient. If one is convinced that unusual fluid deficits are not present and if the hemodynamic and biochemical state of the patient are normal, the use of diuretics is to be preferred. An appropriate regime would be the administration of a bolus of 12.5 gm of mannitol. This will produce an adequate urinary output in most cases. If diuresis does not occur, 50 mg of ethacrynic acid or 40 mg of furosemide should then be given intravenously. It should be remembered that urine volumes in excess of 30 to 50 ml/hr should be replaced by 0.45 per cent sodium chloride solution. In those patients with decreased renal function by preoperative clearance measurements, the prophylactic administration of ethacrynic acid or furosemide is indicated.

POSTOPERATIVE CARE

The maintenance of normal fluid dynamics in the postoperative period prior to the resumption of normal oral intake requires an accurate appraisal of the patient's condition at the close of the operative procedure, a knowledge of the maintenance requirements of the patient under normal conditions and in an average environment, and a precise knowledge of the volume and composition of abnormal losses. A fluid balance record is clearly needed. Daily weights are important. Deficits following the operative procedure should be replaced.

Maintenance requirements for a 70-kg adult will approximate the following:

Volume

Volume of normal fluids should average 2000 to 2500 ml/24 hr. This allows approximately 1000 to 1500 ml for urinary excretion. With this urine volume, the kidney can excrete the estimated load of 300 to 500 milliosmoles of solute per 24 hr at an osmolarity approximating that of the plasma, thus requiring less tubular work for water resorption or water excretion. It should be emphasized that abnormal antidiuretic hormone secretion will probably be present in most postoperative patients for at least a few days and water retention with hypotonicity may occur. The overadministration of electrolyte-free water should be avoided.

Electrolytes

Sodium needs can be satisfied in a patient with relatively good kidney function by the administration of 75 to 100 mEq of sodium per day. Potassium needs can be satisfied by the administration of 20 to 40 mEq per day. Adequate chloride will be administered if sodium and potassium are given as Ringer's lactate with added potassium chloride.

Renal conservation of most electrolytes other than sodium, potassium, and chloride, is adequate to maintain body stores for considerable periods of time in the absence of normal intake. It may be necessary, however, to administer magnesium in small amounts. Magnesium deficiency can occur, especially in the presence of malfunction of the gastrointestinal tract or chronic diarrheal disease [6-120, 6-121]. Replacement may be accomplished by the use of intravenous magnesium sulfate. One milliliter of the 50 per cent magnesium sulfate solution contains 4.1 mEq of magnesium. This may be infused as fast as 0.5 mEq/kg body weight/hr if needed [6-122]. Satisfactory administration of other trace elements can be accomplished by giving the patient one unit of fresh frozen plasma every five to seven days if total intravenous support is required for a long period of time.

Calories

Caloric intake will be below caloric needs, but satisfactory for a few days in the normal individual if at least 100 gm of glucose are administered every 24 hours. This amount will exert the "protein sparing" effect and protect endogenous tissue to a reasonable degree. If parenteral support must be continued for more than a few days, consideration should be given to supplying adequate calories by intravenous alimentation, and attention should be paid to the adequacy of other ions, especially calcium and magnesium.

Abnormal Losses

Abnormal losses should be measured. If these losses are large or continuing, an aliquot of collected drainage should be sent for electrolyte determination. In general, losses of mixed intestinal secretion, whether removed by nasogastric tube or from an ileostomy or fistula, and losses of bile can be replaced with isotonic solutions, usually Ringer's lactate. If the gastric aspirate contains mixed gastric and intestinal secretions, Ringer's lactate may be used. If the aspirate contains only gastric secretion, as with pyloric obstruction, the patient should be treated for the loss of hydrogen and chloride. Measurment of electrolyte concentration in the aspirate should be done in most cases.

During the period of parenteral support, daily urine outputs should be maintained at 1000 to 1500 ml, and measurements of serum electrolytes and creatinine or urea nitrogen should be done to assess the adequacy of treatment and to assure that renal function is maintained.

METABOLIC ALKALOSIS

Alkalosis occurs when excess acid is lost from the organism or excess base added. Virtually the only time this condition is encountered is in a patient where acid gastric content has been lost due to vomiting or protracted nasogastric suction.

The ease and rapidity with which metabolic alkalosis can develop must always be kept in mind. The aspiration of as little as 2.5 to 3 liters of gastric content without appropriate replacement can produce serious distortions in chemical composition when the content has a high concentration of acid [6-123]. An understanding of the pathophysiology of the development of metabolic alkalosis and a clear concept of appropriate therapy is of utmost importance.

Chemical Disturbances

It was recognized in the 1920's that the basic disturbance in this chemical abnormality was the loss of chloride in excess of sodium and potassium, and in terms of acid-base balance, the loss of hydrogen ion in combination with this chloride [6-124, 6-125]. Analysis of the gastric aspirate in patients developing the syndrome shows that chloride is present in a concentration of 90 to 100 mEq/liter, sodium in a concentration of 20 to 40 mEq/liter, and potassium in a concentration of 8 to 10 mEq/liter. As chloride is lost, the anionic gap is made up with bicarbonate and serum bicarbonate levels rise. In patients with vomiting there is always an associated overall decrease in extracellular fluid volume, while in patients where volume replacement has been adequate, the distortion may only be in the composition of the electrolyte rather than in total volume.

Respiratory Response

In contrast to the condition of metabolic acidosis where respiratory compensation to correct blood pH occurs early and is reasonably effective, there is no respiratory compensation to metabolic alkalosis and the P_{CO_2} does not increase [6-126]. Extracellular fluid pH, therefore, rises due to an uncompensated increase in bicarbonate content. The sodium level will be normal or slightly low, potassium normal to low, chloride moderately to severely depressed with values as low as 39 mEq/liter having been recorded, and bicarbonate as high as 40 to 50 mEq/liter [6-126].

Cellular Response

It has been generally agreed that intracellular alterations take place due to transmembrane exchange. A decrease in cell water of 2 to 3 per cent, a decrease in chloride, a decrease in cell potassium, and an increase in cell sodium have been measured by muscle analysis [6-123]. Increase in cell hydrogen ion with a fall in cell pH is said to occur [6-127], although intracellular acidosis may be more directly related to the potassium deficiency per se.

Starvation Effects

Most patients with severe metabolic alkalosis due to loss of gastric secretions are starving due to lack of caloric intake. In these patients, tissue catabolism continues with the liberation of large amounts of potassium into the extracellular fluid. This potassium is then excreted by the kidney. Although total exchangeable potassium decreases, potassium deficiency may not be present. In such situations, intracellular electrolyte and pH levels have been reported to be normal [6-128]. This observation fits well with the clinical experience that patients with relatively severe metabolic alkalosis may show very little disturbance in physiological function over long periods of time providing adequate extracellular volume is maintained.

Renal Effects

The renal effects of metabolic alkalosis are most important in perpetuating the syndrome. In the initial stages, bicarbonate excretion increases and the urine becomes alkaline. As alkalosis and extracellular fluid volume depletion progress, however, several factors come into play to prevent bicarbonate excretion by the kidney and thus reinforce the alkalotic state.

It has been shown that a decrease in extracellular fluid volume alone can interfere with bicarbonate excretion [6-129]. Improvement in renal chloride and hydrogen resorption due to expansion of the extracellular fluid to normal may reverse the alkalosis [6-130]. If extracellular fluid and sodium deficit persist, aldosterone release is stimulated with increase in sodium resorption and a shift from sodium excretion to the excretion of hydrogen ion with the production of an acid urine [6-131].

The major deficiency in renal function has been postulated by Schwartz to be due to the large gap between sodium and chloride levels. Normally the sodium-chloride gap is 35 to 40 mEq. In hypochloremic metabolic alkalosis this gap may increase to 60 to 70 mEq. Schwartz has suggested that isotonic sodium chloride resorption is decreased proportionately as the sodium chloride gap increases, leaving more sodium free for exchange with hydrogen and potassium. In conditions of absolute sodium deficiency and relative potassium deficiency, hydrogen ion is excreted, blocking the excretion of bicarbonate [6-132].

The pH of the urine can be used as a rough guide as to the severity of metabolic alkalosis, with an alkaline or neutral urine indicating early phases and an acid urine indicating a more severe deficiency. Larger losses of sodium have been shown to be associated with the acid urine state [6-126].

Therapy

Treatment of the condition must take into account the primary deficit of chloride ion, hydrogen ion, and volume, with lesser degrees of deficit of sodium ion and perhaps very little actual potassium depletion. It is now clear that correction of the abnormality requires the administration of chloride to replace that deficit, and the administration of potassium alone will not alter the condition [6-133]. Therapy must therefore be begun with two aims in mind. First, replacement of extracellular fluid volume deficits to restore normal hydration. This must be accomplished with sodium chloride solutions, since there is a real sodium deficit. Ringer's lactate should not be used under these conditions, since the extra chloride in sodium chloride is needed. The administration of isotonic sodium chloride alone, however will not correct the alkalosis because the sodium chloride gap is not altered.

If an attempt is made to replace the entire chloride deficit by sodium chloride solutions, hypernatremia with levels up to 160 to 170 mEq/liter will result, and alkalosis will continue due to the large sodium chloride gap. Chloride coupled with some other cation must therefore be administered. Potassium chloride can be used in relatively large amounts, up to 150 to 200 mEq/24 hr (10 mEq/hr). The major effect of this is to replace chloride ion and balance studies have shown that most of the potassium is excreted in the urine. In severe cases, the administration of ammonium chloride will prove effective. The suggestion has been made that replacement of the original deficit be tried, namely the use of 0.15 N hydrochloric acid intravenously [6-134]. This therapy would appear to have some risks and has not been reported frequently in the literature. In severe cases of refractory hypochloremia and alkalosis, hemodialysis should be used. Restoration of a normal electrolyte pattern can usually be achieved by this means.

HYPEROSMOLAR COMA

Decompensation of the regulatory mechanisms which maintain normal osmolarity of the body fluids may occur. The sudden occurrence of a hyperosmolar state in the nonketotic patient was first described in 1951 [6-135]. By 1965 five cases had been reported [6-136]. Since then, however, the syndrome has been seen with increasing frequency—perhaps, paradoxically, because of improved survival of the seriously ill, plus the use of intravenous nutrition including large amounts of glucose.

The syndrome can occur in any patient who is under severe and prolonged stress. In many patients, overt or latent diabetes mellitus is present, but the syndrome has occurred in nondiabetic patients. Moderate to severe renal disease is also frequently seen. In almost all patients large amounts of glucose have been administered.

Clinical Picture

The condition is characterized by the relatively sudden onset (over one to two days) of dehydration, hyperglycemia (often greater than 1000 mg %), hypernatremia, hyperchloremia, and coma. Glycosuria is usually present. Serum potassium is usually within the normal range or low. Ketone bodies and acidosis are absent [6-137].

Effect of Plasma Hyperosmolarity

Plasma osmolarity may rise to 400 to 450 milliosmoles/liter (normal 285 ± 12 milliosmoles/liter). Since extracellular osmolarity is markedly elevated, intracellular dehydration occurs in all tissues. Generalized dehydration occurs also due to the diuretic effect of glycosuria. However, the most severe dehydration occurs in the brain. Water is drawn more strongly from brain cells due to the fact that the blood-brain barrier is impermeable to glucose, with intensification of its osmotic effect [6-138].

In addition to coma due to intracellular dehydration in brain cells, shrinkage of the brain may cause rupture of subarachnoid vessels with hemorrhage and death. Increase in plasma osmolarity may also favor blood coagulation. Disseminated intravascular coagulation has been seen in hyperosmolar coma.

Etiology

The exact cause of the metabolic derangement is obscure. Large amounts of glucose (up to 300 gm/24 hr) may be excreted. This is more than can be mobilized from endogenous glycogen stores and perhaps more than can be created by gluconeogenesis from body proteins. Much of this glucose appears to come from that administered to the patient [6-136].

The absence of ketosis indicates that sufficient insulin activity is present to allow metabolism of enough glucose to provide for basal cell energy needs. However, insulin secretion may be deficient in conditions of prolonged stress [6-139]. The "diabetogenic" effects of stress due to increase in adrenal cortical secretion may play a part in this syndrome. Elevated levels of 17-hydroxycorticoid and cortisol have been measured in such patients [6-136].

Elevation of the blood urea nitrogen is also frequently seen, partially as a result of dehydration, but in many cases caused by defects in renal function. GFR is reduced and tubular function may be altered. One of the puzzling aspects of this syndrome is failure of the water-retention mechanism of the renal tubule. It may be that the osmotic load being excreted by the kidney is so great that water excretion is obligatory. Tubular cell damage may occur because of intensification of the hyperosmolarity of the renal medulla. Tubular cells depend on glycolysis for energy, and glucose entry into these cells may be interfered with. Antidiuretic-hormone levels have not been measured during hyperglycemic diuresis, but it may be that they are not elevated by the hyperglycemia. The injection of hypertonic glucose into the third ventricle of an experimental animal does not produce an antidiuretic hormone response [6-140]. In addition, renal responses to exogenous vasopressin seem somewhat blunted in conditions of hyperosmolar coma.

Diagnosis

The possible occurrence of this syndrome in any severely stressed patient must be kept in mind. The diagnosis has been missed for many days in some patients due to the fact that acidosis is absent so that the usual compensatory mechanisms such as hyperventilation do not occur. Dehydration may be insidious and coma may occur slowly. The occurrence of a urinary output larger than the intake should be a warning signal. Mild degrees of hyperglycemia and persistent glycosuria are also suggestive. Measurement of the blood chemical values makes a positive diagnosis.

The osmolarity of the serum can be measured using the freezing point depression method or calculated using the following formula:

$$\text{Osmolarity} = 2(Na + K) + \frac{mg \% \text{ glucose}}{18} + \frac{mg \% \text{ BUN}}{2.8}$$

Treatment

Therapy is based upon reduction of the hyperglycemia and correction of the dehydration by the administration of hypotonic solutions to return osmolarity to normal. Large amounts of hypotonic fluid may be needed and as much as 17 liters has been administered within a 36-hr period to such a patient [6-141]. Insulin must be given in amounts sufficient to correct the elevated sugar level and potassium supplements are usually required [6-142]. In some cases this therapy will not suffice and the hyperosmolar state will continue. The prompt use of hemodialysis in such refractory conditions will return blood osmolarity and electrolyte levels toward normal. Hemodialysis should be used early to prevent permanent brain damage.

REFERENCES

6-1. Edelman, I. S., Haley, H. B., Schloerb, P. R., Sheldon, D. B., Friis-Hansen, B. J., Stoll, G., and Moore, F. D.: Further observations on total body water. I. Normal values throughout the life span. Surg. Gynec. Obst. 95:1, 1952.

6-2. Wasserman, K., and Mayerson, H. S.: Exchange of albumin between plasma and lymph. Am. J. Physiol. 165:15, 1951.

6-3. Sterling, K.: The turnover rate of serum albumin in man as measured by I^{131}-tagged albumin. J. Clin. Invest. 30:1228, 1951.

6-4. Yoffee, J. M., and Cowtice, F. C.: Lymphatics, lymph and lymphoid tissue. London, Arnold, 1956.

6.5. Berendsen, H. J. C.: Water structure in biological systems. Fed. Proc. 25:971, 1966.

6-6. Berendsen, H. J. C., and Migchelsen, C.: Hydration structure of fibrous macromolecules. Ann. N.Y. Acad. Sci. 125:365, 1965.

6-7.   Ling, G. N.: All-or-none adsorption by living cells and model protein-water systems: discussion of the problem of "permease-induction" and determination of secondary and tertiary structures of proteins. Fed. Proc. 25:958, 1966.

6-8.   Berendsen, H. J. C., and Migchelsen, C.: Hydration structure of collagen and influence of salts. Fed. Proc. 25:998, 1966.

6-9.   Horowitz, S. B., and Fenichel, I. R.: Diffusion and the transport of organic nonelectrolytes in cells. Ann. N.Y. Acad. Sci. 125:572, 1965.

6-10. Gersh, I., and Catchpole, H. R.: The organization of ground substance and basement membrane and its significance in tissue injury, disease and growth. Am. J. Anat. 85:457, 1949.

6-11. Wiederhielm, C. A.: Transcapillary and interstitial transport phenomena in the mesentery. Fed. Proc. 25:1789, 1966.

6-12. Crosti, P., Catchpole, H. R., and Pirani, C. L.: Serum proteins and glycoproteins in papain-injected rabbits. Am. J. Path. 43:419, 1963.

6-13. Begg, T. B., and Hearns, J. B.: Components in blood viscosity. The relative contribution of haematocrit, plasma fibrinogen and other proteins. Clin. Sci. 31:87, 1966.

6-14. Litwin, M. S., Chapman, K., and Stoliar, J. B.: Blood viscosity in the normal man. Surgery 67:342, 1970.

6-15. Putnam, T. C., Kevy, S. V., and Replogle, R. L.: Factors influencing the viscosity of blood. Surg. Gynec. Obst. 124:547, 1967.

6-16. Lee, R. E.: Anatomical and physiological aspects of the capillary bed in the bulbar conjunctiva of man in health and disease. Angiology 6:369, 1955.

6-17. Wells, R. E., Jr., and Merrill, E. W.: Influence of flow properties of blood upon viscosity-hematocrit relationships. J. Clin. Invest. 41:1591, 1962.

6-18. Guyton, A. C., and Richardson, T. Q.: Effect of hematocrit on venous return. Circ. Res. 9:157, 1961.

6-19. Bergentz, S. E., Gelin, L. E., Rudenstam, C.-M., and Zederceldt, B.: The viscosity of whole blood in trauma. Acta Chir. Scand. 126:289, 1963.

6-20   Gelin, L. E.: Disturbance of the flow properties of blood and its counteraction in surgery. Acta Chir. Scand. 122:287, 1961.

6-21. Ditenfass, L.: Viscosity and clotting of blood in venous thrombosis and coronary occlusions. Circ. Res. 14:1, 1964.

6-22. Yao, S. T., and Shoemaker, W. C.: Plasma and whole blood viscosity changes in shock and after dextran infusion. Ann. Surg. 164:973, 1966.

6-23. Murray, J. F., Gold, P., and Johnson, B. L., Jr.: The circulatory effects of hematocrit variations in normovolemic and hypervolemic dogs. J. Clin. Invest. 42:1150, 1963.

6-24. Miller, L. D., Oski, F. A., Diaco, J. F., Sugerman, H. J., Gottlieb, A. J., Davidson, D., and Delivoria-Papadopoulos, M.: The affinity of hemoglobin for oxygen: Its control and in vivo significance. Surgery 68:187, 1970.

6-25. Travis, S. F., Sugerman, H. J., Ruberg, R. L., Dudrick, S. J., Delivoria-Papadopoulos, M., Miller, L. D., and Oski, F. A.: Alterations of red-cell glycolytic intermediates and oxygen transport as a consequence of hypophosphatemia in patients receiving intravenous hyperalimentation. New Engl. J. Med. 285:763, 1971.

6-26. Bunn, H. F., and Jandl, J. H.: Control of hemoglobin function within the red cell. New Engl. J. Med. 282:1414, 1970.

6-27. Valeri, C. R., and Fortier, N. L.: Red-cell 2,3-diphosphoglycerate and creatine levels in patients with red-cell mass deficits or with cardiopulmonary insufficiency. New Engl. J. Med. 281:1452, 1969.

6-28. Miller, L. D., Sugerman, H. J., Miller, W. W., Delivoria-Papadopoulos, M., Diaco, J. F., Gottlieb, A. J., and Oski, F. A.: Increased peripheral oxygen delivery in thyrotoxicosis: Role of red cell 2,3-diphosphoglycerate. Ann. Surg. 172:1058, 1970.

6-29. McCann, R., and DelGuercio, L. R. M.: Respiratory function of blood in the acutely ill patient and the effect of steroids. Ann. Surg. 174:436, 1971.

6-30. Rodriguez, J. M., and Shahidi, N. T.: Erythrocyte 2,3-diphosphoglycerate in adaptive red-cell-volume deficiency. New Engl. J. Med. 285:479, 1971.

6-31. Bunn, H. F., May, M. H., Kocholaty, W. F., and Shields, C. E.: Hemoglobin function in stored blood. J. Clin. Invest. 48:311, 1969.

6-32. Moore, F. D.: The effects of hemorrhage on body composition. New Engl. J. Med. 273:567, 1965.

6-33. Skillman, J. J., Awwad, H. K., and Moore, F. D.: Plasma protein kinetics of the early transcapillary refill after hemorrhage in man. Surg. Gynec. Obst. 125:983, 1967.

6-34. Cope, O., and Litwin, S. B.: Contribution of the lymphatic system to the replenishment of the plasma volume following a hemorrhage. Ann. Surg. 156:655, 1962.

6-35. Adamson, J., and Hillman, R. S.: Blood volume and plasma protein replacement following acute blood loss in normal man. JAMA 205:609, 1968.

6-36. Wilson, R. F., Bassett, J. S., and Walt, A. J.: Five years of experience with massive blood transfusions. JAMA 194:851, 1965.

6-37. Boyan, C. P.: Cold or warmed blood for massive transfusions. Ann. Surg. 160:282, 1964.

6-38. Schechter, D. C., and Swan, H.: Biochemical alterations of preserved blood. Results in two different citrate solutions (ACD and CPD). Arch. Surg. 84:269, 1962.

6-39. Howland, W. S., Schweizer, O., and Boyan, C. P.: The effect of buffering on the mortality of massive blood replacement. Surg. Gynec. Obst. 121:777, 1965.

6-40. Miller, R. D., Tong, M. J., and Robbins, T. O.: Effects of massive transfusion of blood on acid-base balance. JAMA 216:1762, 1971.

6-41. Bunker, J. P., Bendixen, H. H., and Murphy, A. J.: Hemodynamic effects of intravenously administered sodium citrate. New Engl. J. Med. 266:372, 1962.

6-42. Howland, W. S., Schweizer, O., and Boyan, C. P.: Massive blood replacement without calcium administration. Surg. Gynec. Obst. 118:814, 1964.

6-43. Krevans, J. R., and Jackson, D. P.: Hemorrhagic disorder following massive whole blood transfusions. JAMA 159:171, 1955.

6-44. Simmons, R. L., Collins, J. A., Heisterkamp, C. A., III, Mills, D. E., Andren, R., and Phillips, L. L.: Coagulation disorders in combat casualties. I. Acute changes after wounding. II. Effects of massive transfusion. III. Post-resuscitative changes. Ann. Surg. 169: 455, 1969.

6-45. Allen, J. C., and Kunkel, H. G.: Antibodies against gamma globulin after repeated blood transfusions in man. J. Clin. Invest. 45:29, 1966.

6-46. Chaplin, H., Jr.: Current concepts. Packed red blood cells. New Engl. J. Med. 281:364, 1969.

6-47. Huggins, C. E.: Frozen blood. Ann. Surg. 160:643, 1964.

6-48. Moss, G. S., Naleri, C. R., and Brodine, C. E.: Clinical experience with the use of frozen blood in combat casualties. New Engl. J. Med. 278:748, 1968.

6-49. Yudin, S. S.: Transfusion of stored cadaver blood: Practical considerations: First 1000 cases. Lancet. 2:361, 1937.

6-50. Moore, C. L., Pruitt, J. C., and Meredith, J. H.: Present status of cadaver blood as transfusion medium. Arch. Surg. 85:364, 1962.

6-51. Milles, G., Langston, H., and Dalessandro, W.: Experiences with autotransfusions. Surg. Gynec. Obst. 115:689, 1962.

6-52. Langston, H. T., Milles, G., and Dalessandro, W.: Further experiences with autogenous blood transfusions. Ann. Surg. 158: 333, 1963.

6-53. Wilson, J. D., and Taswell, H. F.: Autotransfusion: Historical review and preliminary report on a new method. Mayo Clin. Proc. 43:26, 1968.

6-54. Berlin, N. I.: Determination of red blood cell life span. JAMA 188:375, 1964.

6-55. Haynes, L. L., Turville, W. C., Sproul, M. T., Henderson, M. E., Zemp, J. W., and Tullis, J. L.: Long-term blood preservation—a reality. J. Mich. St. Med. Soc. 61:1509, 1962.

6-56. Rabner, S. F., O'Brien, K., Peskin, G. W., and Friedman, L. H.:
       Further studies with stroma-free hemoglobin solution. Ann. Surg.
       171:615, 1970.

6-57. Geyer, R. P.: Whole animal perfusion with fluorocarbon disper-
       sions. Fed. Proc. 29:1758, 1970.

6-58. Hegarty, J. C., and Stahl, W. M.: Homologous blood syndrome. J.
       Thorac. Cardiovasc. Surg. 53:415, 1967.

6-59. Gruber, U. F., and Bergentz, S. E.: Autologous and homologous
       fresh human plasma as a volume expander in hypovolemic sub-
       jects. Ann. Surg. 165:41, 1967.

6-60. McNamara, J. J., Boatright, D., Burran, E. L., Molot, M. D.,
       Summers, E., and Stremple, J. F.: Changes in some physical
       properties of stored blood. Ann. Surg. 174:58, 1971.

6-61. Rush, B. F., Jr., Richardson, J. D., Bosomworth, P., and Eise-
       man, B.: Limitations of blood replacement with electrolyte solu-
       tions. A controlled clinical study. Arch. Surg. 98:49, 1969.

6-62. Cloutier, C. T., Lowery, B. D., and Carey, L. C.: The effect of
       hemodilutional resuscitation on serum protein levels in humans
       in hemorrhagic shock. J. Trauma 9:514, 1969.

6-63. Baue, A. E., Tragus, E. T., Wolfson, S. K., Cary, A. L., and
       Parkins, W. M.: Hemodynamic and metabolic effects of Ringer's
       lactate solution in hemorrhagic shock. Ann. Surg. 166:29,
       1967.

6-64. Moss, G. S., Proctor, H. J., Homer, L. D., Herman, C. M., and
       Litt, B. D.: A comparison of asanguineous fluids and whole
       blood in the treatment of hemorrhagic shock Surg. Gynec. Obst.
       129:1247, 1969.

6-65. Takaori, M., and Safar, P.: Treatment of massive hemorrhage with
       colloid and crystalloid solutions. Studies in dogs. JAMA 199:297,
       1967.

6-66. Golub, S., Vanichanan, C., Schaefer, C., and Schechter, D. C.: A
       study of safer plasma substitutes. Surg. Gynec. Obst. 128:1235,
       1968.

6-67. Marty, A. T., and Zweifach, B. W.: The high oncotic pressure
       effects of dextrans. Arch. Surg. 101:421, 1970.

6-68. Atik, M..: The use of dextran in surgery: A current evaluation.
       Surgery 65:548, 1969.

6-69. Schwartz, S. I., Shay, H. P., Beebe, H., and Rob, C.: Effect of
       low molecular weight dextran on venous flow. Surgery 55:106,
       1964.

6-70. Folse, R., and Cope, J. G.: A comparison of the peripheral and
       central hemodynamic effects of regular and low molecular
       weight dextran in patients with ischemic limbs. Surgery 58:779,
       1965.

6-71. George, J. N., and Breckenridge, R. T.: The use of factor VIII and
       factor IX concentrates during surgery. JAMA 214:1673, 1970.

6-72. Britten, A. F. H., and Salzman, E. W.: Surgery in congenital disorders of blood coagulation. Surg. Gynec. Obst. 123:1333, 1966.

6-73. Attar, S., Boyd, D., Layne, E., McLaughlin, J., Mansberger, A. R., and Cowley, R. A.: Alterations in coagulation and fibrinolytic mechanisms in acute trauma. J. Trauma 9:939, 1969.

6-74. Borowiecki, B., and Sharp, A. A.: Trauma and fibrinolysis. J. Trauma 9:522, 1969.

6-75. Crowell, J. W., and Read, W. L.: In vivo coagulation—a probable cause of irreversible shock. Am. J. Physiol. 183:566, 1955.

6-76. Hardaway, R. M., and Weiss, F. H.: Intracapillary clotting as the etiology of shock. Arch. Surg. 83:851, 1961.

6-77. Hardaway, R. M.: The role of intravascular clotting in the etiology of shock. Ann. Surg. 155:325, 1962.

6-78. String, T., Robinson, A. J., and Blaisdell, F. W.: Massive trauma. Effect of intravascular coagulation on prognosis. Arch. Surg. 92:406, 1971.

6-79. Corrigan, J. J., Jr., Ray, W. L., and May, N.: Changes in the blood coagulation system associated with septicemia. New Engl. J. Med. 279:851, 1968.

6-80. Rodriguez-Erdmann, F.: Bleeding due to increased intravascular blood coagulation. Hemorrhagic syndromes caused by consumption of blood-clotting factors (consumption-coagulopathies). New Engl. J. Med. 273:1370, 1965.

6-81. Pechet, L.: Fibrinolysis (Concluded). New Engl. J. Med. 273:1024, 1965.

6-82. Zweifach, B. W.: The microcirculation of the blood. Sci. Am. 200:54, 1959.

6-83. Guyton, A. C., and Coleman, T. G.: Regulation of interstitial fluid volume and pressure. Ann. N.Y. Acad. Sci. 150:537, 1968.

6-84. Burgen, A. S. V., and Francombe, W. H.: The role of plasma colloid osmotic pressure in the regulation of extracellular fluid. Proc. International Union Physiol. Sci., XXII Internat. Cong., Leiden, 2:130, 1962.

6-85. Guyton, A. C.: A concept of negative interstitial pressure based on pressures in implanted perforated capsules. Circ. Res. 12:399, 1963.

6-86. Mayerson, H. S.: On lymph and lymphatics. Circulation 28:839, 1963.

6-87. Drinker, C. K.: he lymphatic system. Lane Medical Series, Stanford Univ. Press, Stanford, Calif., 1942.

6-88. Hall, J. G., Morris, B., and Woolley, G.: Intrinsic rhythmic propulsion of lymph in the unanaesthetized sheep. J. Physiol. 180:336, 1965.

6-89. Majno, G., Gilmore, V., and Leventhal, M.: On the mechanism of vascular leakage caused by histamine-type mediators. A microscopic study in vivo. Circ. Res. 21:833, 1967.

6-90. Hendley, E. D., and Schiller, A. A.: Change in capillary permeability during hypoxemic perfusion of rat hindlegs. Am. J. Physiol. 179:216, 1954.

6-91. Warren, M. F., and Drinker, C. K.: The flow of lymph from the lungs of the dog. Am. J. Physiol. 136:207, 1942.

6-92. Strock, P. E.: Microvascular changes in acutely ischemic rat muscle. Surg. Gynec. Obst. 129:1213, 1969.

6-93. Chien, S., Sinclair, D. G., Dellenback, R. J., Chang, C., Peric, B., Usami, S., and Gregersen, M. I.: Effect of endotoxin on capillary permeability to macromolecules. Am. J. Physiol. 207:518, 1964.

6-94. Arturson, G.: Pathophysiological aspects of the burn syndrome. Acta Chir. Scand. Suppl. 274:1, 1961.

6-95. Tosteson, D. C.: Symposium on the molecular basis of membrane function. Englewood Cliffs, N.J., Prentice-Hall, 1969.

6-96. Whittam, R.: Transport and diffusion in red blood cells. Baltimore, Williams & Wilkins, 1964.

6-97. Leaf, A.: On the mechanism of fluid exchange of tissues in vitro. Biochem. J. 62:241, 1956.

6-98. Ege, R., Gottlieb, E., and Rakestraw, N. W.: The distribution of glucose between human blood plasma and red corpuscles and the rapidity of its penetration. Am. J. Physiol. 72:76, 1925.

6-99. Enerson, D. M., and Berman, H. M.: Cellular swelling II: Effects of hypotonicity, low molecular weight dextran addition and pH changes on oxygen consumption of isolated tissues. Ann. Surg. 163:537, 1966.

6-100. Wacker, W. E. C.: The biochemistry of magnesium. Ann. N.Y. Acad. Sci. 162:717, 1969.

6-101. Henzel, J. H., DeWeese, M. S., and Pories, W. J.: Significance of magnesium and zinc metabolism in the surgical patient. II. Zinc. Arch. Surg. 95:991, 1967.

6-102. Westmorland, N.: Connective tissue alterations in zinc deficiency. Fed. Proc. 30:1001, 1971.

6-103. Leach, R. M., Jr.: Role of manganese in mucopolysaccharide metabolism. Fed. Proc. 30:991, 1971.

6-104. Cornes, W. H.: Role of copper in connective tissue metabolism. Fed. Proc. 30:995, 1971.

6-105. McCall, J. T., Goldstein, N. P., and Smith, L. H.: Implications of trace metals in human diseases. Fed. Proc. 30:1011, 1971.

6-106. Schroeder, H. A., and Balassa, J. J.: Abnormal trace metals in man: Cadmium, J. Chronic Dis. 14:236, 1961.

6-107. O'Shaughnessy, W. B.: Experiments on the blood in cholera. Lancet 1:410, 1831.

6-108. Latta, T.: Malignant cholera. Lancet 2:274, 1832.

6-109. Coller, F. A., and Maddock, W. G.: A study of dehydration in humans. Ann. Surg. 102:947, 1935.

6-110. Lapides, J., Bourne, R. B., and MacLean, L. R.: Clinical signs of dehydration and extracellular fluid loss. JAMA 191:413, 1965.

6-111. Billig, D. M., and Jordan, P. H., Jr.: Hemodynamic abnormalities secondary to extracellular fluid depletion in intestinal obstruction. Surg. Gynec. Obst. 128:1274, 1969.

6-112. Shires, T., Williams, J., and Brown, F.: Acute change in extracellular fluids associated with major surgical procedures. Ann. Surg. 154:803, 1961.

6-113. Gilder, H., Cortese, A. F., Loehr, W. J., Moore, H. V., and deLeon, V.: Dilution studies in experimental hemorrhagic and endotoxic shock. A critical look at the excessive deficits of extracellular space in shocked dogs. Ann. Surg. 171:42, 1970.

6-114. Crystal, R. B., and Baue, A. E.: Influence of hemorrhagic hypotension on measurements of the extracellular fluid volume. Surg. Gynec. Obst. 129:576, 1969.

6-115. Anderson, R. W., Simmons, R. L., Collins, J. A., Bredenberg, C. E., James, P. M., and Levitsky, S.: Plasma volume and sulfate spaces in acute combat casualties. Surg. Gynec. Obst. 128:719, 1969.

6-116. Fountain, S. S., and Schloerb, P. R.: The dynamics of posttraumatic intestinal fluid sequestration. Surg. Gynec. Obst. 123:1237, 1966.

6-117. Hoye, R. C., Paulson, D. F., and Ketcham, A. S.: Total circulating albumin deficits occurring with extensive surgical procedures. Surg. Gynec. Obst. 131:943, 1970.

6-118. Hoye, R. C., and Ketcham, A. S.: Shifts in body fluids during radical surgery. Cancer 20:1827, 1967.

6-119. Stahl, W. M.: Intra-operative volume support by sodium infusion: an approach to quantitation. Surg. Forum. 18:30, 1967.

6-120. Wacker, W. E. C., and Parisis, A. F.: Magnesium metabolism. New Engl. J. Med. 278:712, 1968.

6-121. Heaton, F. W., Clark, C. G., and Goligher, J. C.: Magnesium deficiency complicating intestinal surgery. Brit. J. Surg. 54:41, 1967.

6-122. Henzel, J. H., DeWeese, M. S., and Ridenhour, G.: Significance of magnesium and zinc metabolism in the surgical patient. I. Magnesium. Arch. Surg. 95:974, 1967.

6-123. Ariel, I. M.: The effects of acute hypochloremia on the distribution of body fluid and composition of tissue electrolytes in man. Ann. Surg. 140:150, 1954.

6-124. MacCallum, W. G., Lintz, J., Vermilye, H. N., Leggett, T. H., and Boas, E.: The effect of pyloric obstruction in relation to gastric tetany. Johns Hopkins Hosp. Bull. 31:1, 1920.

6-125. Gamble, J. L., and Ross, S. G.: The factors in the dehydration following pyloric obstruction. J. Clin. Invest. 1:403, 1925.

6-126. Howe, C. T., and LeQuesne, L. P.: Pyloric stenosis: The metabolic effects. Brit. J. Surg. 51:923, 1964.

6-127. Irvine, R. O. H., Saunders, S. J., Milne, M. D., and Crawford, M. A.: Gradients of potassium and hydrogen ion in potassium-deficient voluntary muscle. Clin. Sci. 20:1, 1960.

6-128. Schloerb, P. R., and Grantham, J. J.: Intracellular pH and muscle electrolytes in metabolic alkalosis from loss of gastric juice. Surgery 56:144, 1964.

6-129. Kurtzman, N. A.: Regulation of renal bicarbonate reabsorption by extracellular volume. J. Clin. Invest. 49:586, 1970.

6-130. Cohen, J. J.: Correction of metabolic alkalosis by the kidney after isometric expansion of extracellular fluid. J. Clin. Invest. 47:1181, 1968.

6-131. LeQuesne, L. P.: Body fluid disturbance resulting from pyloric dysfunction. Surg. Gynec. Obst. 113:1, 1961.

6-132. Needle, M. A., Kaloyanides, G. J., and Schwartz, W. B.: The effects of selective depletion of hydrochloric acid on acid-base and electrolyte equilibrium. J. Clin. Invest. 43:1836, 1964.

6-133. Atkins, E. L., and Schwartz, W. B.: Factors governing correction of the alkalosis associated with potassium deficiency: The critical role of chloride in the recovery process. J. Clin. Invest. 41:218, 1962.

6-134. Bradham, G. B.: The intravenous use of hydrochloric acid in the treatment of severe alkalosis. Am. Surg. 34:551, 1968.

6-135. Evans, E. I., and Butterfield, W. J. H.: The stress response in the severely burned: An interim report. Ann. Surg. 134:588, 1951.

6-136. Rosenberg, S. A., Brief, D. K., Kinney, J. M., Herrera, M. G., Wilson, R. E., and Moore, F. D.: The syndrome of dehydration, coma and severe hyperglycemia without ketosis in patients convalescing from burns. New Engl. J. Med. 272:931, 1965.

6-137. Danowski, T. S.: Non-ketotic coma and diabetes mellitus. Med. Clin. No. Amer. 55:913, 1971.

6-138. Andersson, B.: Thirst—and brain control of water balance. Am. Sci. 59:408, 1971.

6-139. Seltzer, H. S., and Harris, V. L.: Exhaustion of insulogenic reserve in maturity-onset diabetic patients during prolonged and continuous hyperglycemic stress. Diabetes 13:6, 1964.

6-140. Andersson, B., Olsson, K., and Warner, R. G.: Dissimilarities between the central control of thirst and the release of antidiuretic hormone (ADH) Acta Physiol. Scand. 71:57, 1967.

6-141. Cohen, P. G.: Hyperosmolar coma: A geriatric medical emergency. Geriatrics 25:102, 1970.

6-142. Ashworth, C. J., Jr., Sacks, Y., Williams, L. F., Jr., and Byrne, J. J.: Hyperosmolar hyperglycemic non-ketotic coma: its importance in surgical problems. Ann. Surg. 167:556, 1968.

PART III

Regulatory Systems

7

LIVER

The normal liver is an important chemical regulatory system of the body. Therefore liver cell failure, whether acute or chronic, imposes widespread and complex metabolic disturbances.

THE ANHEPATIC STATE

Sudden removal of the liver in the primate produces cardiovascular and hematologic changes which cause the death of the animal [7-1]. A rapid decline in cardiac output occurs with bradycardia, together with the swift onset of the defibrination syndrome. Blood pressure may be maintained by peripheral constriction for several hours. After this time vasodilatation occurs and shock develops. There is a progressive decline in body temperature, a fall in blood pH, a rapid decrease in serum protein, a fall in serum sodium, and a rise in serum potassium. Tissue perfusion decreases with acidosis and oliguria. An increase in the rate of fall of fibrinogen levels at this late stage suggests that disseminated intravascular coagulation takes place [7-2].

LIVER FUNCTION

Glycogen

The importance of liver glycogen as an available source of glucose and as a stabilizing influence on glucose metabolism has been known

189

for many years. Absence of liver glycogen stores due to preexisting mal-nutrition or severe stress decreases the ability of the liver to release adequate amounts of glucose under new stress. Following massive hepatic resection, hypoglycemia is a constant threat which must be countered by infused glucose [7-3]. In some instances glucose metabolism does not return to normal for one to two weeks following hepatic resection [7-4].

Lipids

Changes in lipid metabolism also occur following massive hepatic resection, with an initial increase in nonesterified fatty acids. This is followed by a decrease to low levels, with return to normal at approximately one week [7-3].

Proteins

Plasma proteins are synthesized in the liver cell. Extensive removal of liver tissue results in a fall in total protein, with a severe decrease in all globulin fractions [7-5]. Decrease in synthesis of a variety of proteins has been shown in patients with hepatocellular disease [7-6]. Albumin synthesis has been studied and is depressed in most patients with acute or chronic hepatocellular disease [7-7]. The hypoalbuminemia of liver failure is due to this decreased synthetic rate coupled with increased intestinal losses and an expanded plasma volume. Albumin catabolism appears to be normal [7-8]. Fibrinogen synthesis also appears to be depressed in patients with liver disease [7-6].

Pigment Excretion

Hepatic cells metabolize, conjugate, and excrete bilirubin and other pigments into the bile. Failure of such metabolism produces a rise in circulating pigment, usually in the unconjugated form. Sulfobromophthalein is conjugated and excreted in a manner similar to bilirubin and forms the basis of the BSP test of pigment excretory function.

Enzyme Excretion

Under normal conditions the liver excretes certain enzymes into the bile. Obstruction of bile flow leads to elevation of serum levels of alkaline phosphatase [7-9, 7-10]. Liver cell damage enhances the release of other intracellular enzymes (transaminases) [7-11]. There is evidence that amylase is also produced by the liver and excreted into the bile [7-12].

Urea Synthesis

Incorporation of aminonitrogen into urea occurs in the liver. If portal blood bypasses the liver through naturally occurring shunts or following the creation of a portosystemic shunt, ammonia levels can rise in the blood. Malfunction of liver cells reduces urea synthesis and allows the blood ammonia to increase. Increase in blood ammonia levels have been implicated as a cause of hepatic encephalopathy, although this relationship is still not clear.

Coagulation Factors

The normal coagulation system depends on the production of several factors by the liver. Patients with diffuse liver damage may have a variety of coagulation defects [7-13]. Factors synthesized in the liver are Factor IIs (prothrombin), V, VII, IX, X, and XIII. Defects in fibrinogen also affect the clotting mechanism. All of these clotting factors are usually depressed collectively as liver function decreases [7-14]. The decrease in levels of Factor V appears to parallel the severity of liver disease, and a fatal outcome is often indicated when Factor V levels fall below 50 per cent [7-15].

Thrombocytopenia and thrombasthenia are frequently seen with liver-cell disease, and thrombocytopenia occurs rapidly after removal of the liver. The exact reasons for this are as yet not known. Fibrinolysis has been suggested as the cause of abnormal bleeding in many patients with hepatic dysfunction [7-13]. This increase in lytic activity may be the result of a decreased synthesis of a lytic inhibitor [7-16].

Hormone Metabolism

Normal liver function also plays an important role in the regulation of endocrine balance. Corticosteroids are metabolized in the liver, the rate of removal increasing as plasma hormone levels rise. The reverse occurs if plasma levels fall, producing a direct regulatory mechanism [7-17]. Decrease in liver function allows corticosteroids to accumulate at a higher level in the blood [7-18]. Accumulation of aldosterone may lead to abnormal sodium and water retention. Lack of metabolism of estrogens may produce gynecomastia in the male.

Vasopressin is cleared by the liver and kidney. When serum vasopressin levels are in the normal range, approximately one-third is cleared by hepatic-cell function. However, in the anesthetized animal, or with abnormally high vasopressin levels, hepatic clearance may reach two-thirds of the total clearance. Hepatic dysfunction, therefore, can decrease the removal of vasopressin from the serum, especially under conditions where vasopressin levels are increased or where renal blood flow is decreased. The danger of water retention and hypotonicity, thus, increases in the patient with hepatic cell dysfunction [7-19].

HEPATITIS

Hepatic cellular dysfunction may be either acute or chronic. Acute liver failure is usually the result of viral hepatitis, or more rarely due to the administration of substances which are hepatotoxic. Viral hepatitis may be transmitted by contact, or by the ingestion of infected foods, often shellfish [7-20], or by the injection of virus through needle penetration of the skin. It is thus frequently seen in drug addicts and in transfused patients who have received infected blood. In the latter group, those patients transfused from commercial donors have a much higher incidence of hepatitis than those transfused from volunteer donors [7-21]. The suggestion has been made that administration of gamma globulin will partially protect against the development of this type of transfusion hepatitis [7-22]. Testing for the presence of Australian antigen will help to screen out infected bloods.

HEPATOTOXINS

Hepatotoxic substances may act through direct injury to liver cells with cell injury being dose related [7-23]. Such substances are carbon tetrachloride, inorganic phosphorus, and poison from the mushroom *Amanita phalloides*. Drugs may also produce damage by indirect means, by blocking metabolic pathways or interfering with bilirubin excretion. Examples of this latter group are the anabolic steroids [7-24].

Drug hepatotoxins commonly encountered in surgical practice include chlorpromazine, which produces jaundice in 1 to 5 per cent of those receiving the drug [7-25]. This substance produces a hepatocanalicular picture with chemical signs of intrahepatic obstruction. Iproniazide, cincophen, phenylbutazone, and propylthiouracil have been shown to produce hepatotoxicity of a cellular type. Antimicrobial agents have been implicated in the production of liver toxicity, especially erythromycin and oleandomycin [7-26]. The production of hepatocellular damage by halothane anesthesia has been reported. This appears to be an idiosyncratic type of reaction and is not dose-related.

CIRRHOSIS

Liver damage of a chronic type is almost always the result of damage to hepatic cells with replacement by fibrosis. Chronic biliary obstruction produces one distinct form of hepatic cell destruction due to ductal pressure and pigment deposition. More commonly hepatic cell damage occurs due to the chronic use of alcohol, or from the acute necrotic changes of viral hepatitis or drug induced hepatic necrosis. The alcoholic and postnecrotic groups of patients present many similarities, but there are differences which must be kept in mind [7-27, 7-28]. The patient with progressive and continuing alcoholism is subject to acute changes in liver function following alcohol intake. Acute hepatic decompensation may occur as shown by jaundice, fever, ascites, and leukocytosis, which however may improve with abstinence from alcohol. In the postnecrotic group or in the alcoholic subject who has abstained from alcohol for many years, the state of liver function is less variable and when signs of deterioration of liver function appear, a progressive downhill course usually follows.

Differentiation of the two types of nonbiliary cirrhosis may be extremely difficult both clinically and pathologically. The fact that more than 50 per cent of patients with postnecrotic cirrhosis also have had a prolonged alcoholic intake confuses the picture. It appears that the postnecrotic patient more often has portal hypertension with splenomegaly, varices, and hemorrhage, whereas the alcoholic patient more often has jaundice and ascites, and less often splenomegaly. The patient with postnecrotic cirrhosis may be able to withstand operation better than the alcoholic patient [7-28].

Alcoholism

Alcoholism per se has generalized effects in addition to the direct hepatotoxic action [7-29]. Malnutrition commonly accompanies chronic alcoholism. It has been shown that subsequent to the ingestion of a standard amount of alcohol, higher blood levels are attained as caloric intake is decreased [7-30]. Alcoholics may thus decrease oral food intake to potentiate the effect of alcohol. This response is apparently due to a slowing of ethanol metabolism by the liver [7-31]. Since operation and anesthesia have been shown to cause an increased liver injury in malnourished patients, alcoholics are at higher risk for further liver damage when operated upon [7-32].

Chronic alcohol ingestion may cause an increased level of catecholamine due to suppression of the sensitivity of receptor sites. In addition, elevated aldosterone levels have been shown with continued ingestion of alcohol [7-33]. Upon cessation of drinking with return of sensitivity of receptor sites, catecholamine response may be exaggerated. This may play a part in the hyperdynamic state of acute alcoholic withdrawal.

HEPATIC EFFECTS OF SHOCK

Liver function is adversely effected by events occurring in shock and trauma. In the presence of hemorrhagic hypotension, liver blood flow falls concomitantly with the fall in cardiac output. Splanchnic blood flow, and thus portal flow, falls to a greater degree than the fall in cardiac output [7-34]. Central liver-cell necrosis has been seen in human shock and apparently is related to the duration of the shock state [7-35]. Animal studies have shown slowing of the microcirculation in the primate liver during shock. Mitochondrial changes have been observed by electron microscopy in the liver cells of shocked rats [7-36, 7-37].

HEPATIC ANOXIA

The effects of hepatic anoxia produced by ligation of the hepatic artery and diversion of portal flow have been studied in animals and have been reported following accidental hepatic artery ligation in man [7-38]. These patients and animals demonstrate hypotension, tachycardia, oliguria, and jaundice with a rise in SGOT (serum glutamic oxaloacetic transaminase) and SGPT (serum glutamic pyruvic transaminase) levels. There is often fever, abdominal distention, and a rising BUN. The patient usually succumbs to "hepatorenal failure" and coma. Following an episode of hepatic anoxia, the degree of elevation of the enzymes

SGOT, SGPT, and LDH (lactic dehydrogenase) seems to parallel the degree of anoxic damage [7-39].

Other results of hepatic anoxia have been discovered during experiences with liver homotransplantation. Acidosis usually occurs following liver revascularization, the severity of which is proportional to the degree of anoxia [7-40]. Uptake of potassium occurs if the ischemic period is short and serious hypokalemia can result. If the ischemic period is prolonged, leakage of potassium from the liver continues and hyperkalemia results. Alterations in fibrinolytic activity are also seen, with increased fibrinolysis present when the liver is anoxic. Levels return to normal if liver survival occurs [7-41].

CHEMICAL SHOCK

Shock due to chemical agents also causes changes in liver function. Endotoxin injection causes an increase in circulating SGOT, SGPT, and alkaline phosphatase [7-42]. Cell damage occurs with depression of mitochondrial respiration [7-43], and leakage of lysosomal enzymes [7-44]. Histologic study of human liver tissue following death from pancreatitis has shown necrosis and bile stasis in 78 per cent of cases [7-45].

EFFECTS OF TRAUMA

Evidence of liver injury has been found following severe systemic trauma [7-46] and following operation [7-32, 7-47]. Improved supportive care and nutrition may reduce the injury to the liver occurring during abdominal operations. A recent study showed elevation in circulating enzymes in only 5 per cent of 56 patients [7-48]. The combination of shock, major operation or injury, and multiple transfusions can produce a syndrome of liver failure with jaundice in the posttrauma period [7-49, 7-50]. The presence of renal failure may also contribute to the picture due to impaired excretion of bilirubin [7-51].

HYPERDYNAMIC CIRCULATORY FAILURE

Failure of normal function of hepatic cells may produce secondary effects in many other organ systems. Alteration in cardiovascular function with systemic and pulmonary shunting has been shown to occur in states of chronic hepatic failure [7-52, 7-53, 7-54]. Cardiac output must rise to maintain pressure and flow in the presence of decreased vascular resistance, and the "hyperdynamic state" results [7-55]. When myocardial reserve is insufficient to maintain the required level of output, decompensation occurs with hypotension and terminal hepatic failure. In such patients, cardiac muscle has been shown to be unresponsive to injected tyramine, suggesting depletion of tissue epinephrine stores [7-56]. This finding is similar to that in experimental heart failure [7-57].

HEPATORENAL SYNDROME

Renal failure and the development of the hepatorenal syndrome may occur in patients with liver decompensation. The exact nature of the renal lesion in this syndrome has been a puzzle for many years, inasmuch as the structure of the kidney by histologic examination has always appeared essentially normal. Koppell and coworkers were able to transplant seven kidneys from patients dying from the hepatorenal syndrome into patients with end-stage renal disease and normal liver function [7-58]. Improvement in renal function occurred in all but one recipient. The functional problem in such kidneys appears to be one of regulation of intrarenal blood flow [7-59]. Epstein et al have reported absence of cortical flow in such patients [7-60]. Renal function may be impaired in patients with cirrhosis because of increase in inferior vena cava pressure [7-61] or increase in intraperitoneal pressure [7-62]. Hypovolemia may be present in such patients and if so fluid infusion improves renal function. However, patients in the hyperdynamic state show little response to any additional volume [7-63].

HEALING AND RESISTANCE TO INFECTION

Hepatic failure causes a decrease in the rate of wound healing and an increased incidence of infection. Such patients have been shown to have deficiencies of alpha, beta, and gamma globulin. Immunoelectrophoresis shows a decrease in 19-S gamma globulin with preservation of 7-S fraction. Inspite of this potential for antibody formation, Norman et al were unable to show the development of any antibody in patients with hepatic failure as long as 18 days after xenogeneic extracorporeal liver perfusion [7-64].

HEPATIC FUNCTION TESTS

It has been shown that an individual may survive the acute removal of up to 90 per cent of a normal liver [7-3], with the remaining 10 per cent having the capability of maintaining life. Transient evidence of hepatic insufficiency occurs but regeneration rapidly returns function to normal. Diffuse liver disease, therefore, must produce functional abnormality in all liver cells, or destruction of a large proportion of normal liver cells, to be detectable by ordinary methods.

The usual tests for pigment metabolism are the measurement of serum bilirubin and the sulfobromophthalein retention test. Protein synthesis can be estimated by measurement of the circulating serum albumin and by protein electrophoresis. Clotting factors can be measured. Evidence of obstructive biliary disease can be obtained by measurement of the alkaline phosphatase, stool and urine bile, and urine urobilinogen. Measurement of the serum level of enzymes, SGOT, SGPT, and LDH indicates the severity and activity of hepatocellular damage.

Evidence of failure of hormone metabolism may be detected by noting the presence of gynecomastia and a feminine hair distribution (estrogens) in the male, sodium retention with edema, ascites, and hypokalemia (aldosterone), excess water retention with hypotonicity (vasopressin). The presence of abnormal vasoactive substances may be suspected by the presence of cutaneous vasodilatation, tachycardia, and hypotension. Arterial and venous blood gases will indicate pulmonary shunting with an increase in the alveolar-arterial oxygen difference, and peripheral shunting with a diminution in the arteriovenous oxygen difference.

PREOPERATIVE EVALUATION

The history should clearly outline any evidence of previous or present liver damage. This will include a history of jaundice, biliary-tract disease, hepatitis, or exposure to hepatotoxic agents. Information as to the general state of well-being is important with regard to strength, energy, muscular atrophy or weight loss, swelling of the abdomen or leg edema, and significant shortness of breath or tachycardia.

The physical examination should be made with care to evaluate skin turgor, hair distribution, presence of cutaneous vasodilatation in the palms or face, presence of spider telangiectasia, hepatosplenomegaly, ascites, jaundice, and ankle edema. Measurement of serum electrolytes, creatinine, BUN, fasting sugar, alkaline phosphatase, bilirubin, SGOT, SGPT, and LDH should be made. Serum albumin and globulin levels should be measured and protein electrophoresis performed. Evidence of the hyperdynamic state should be sought and blood gases measured to confirm pulmonary or peripheral shunting. Exercise tolerance is an important measurement in the patient with liver disease, since it has been shown that survival may depend on the ability of the myocardium to respond to the demands of the systemic shunt [7-53].

Experience in the assessment of patients for portosystemic shunting operations has shown that survival is more commonly associated with reasonable levels of liver function [7-65, 7-66, 7-67]. Such function is measured by a serum albumin of greater than 3 gm/100 ml, the absence of ascites, sulfobromophthalein retention of less than 25 per cent, bilirubin less than 2 mg %, and prothrombin content greater than 50 per cent of normal. Absence of pulmonary shunting as evidenced by a normal arterial oxygen level and a good response to exercise testing are additional indications that the patient will survive operation. If chemical factors are not in this relatively acceptable range, and if evidence of pulmonary and systemic shunting is present, with poor response to exercise, the risk of operation, especially the performance of a portosystemic shunt, may be prohibitive.

PREOPERATIVE PREPARATION

The intent is to optimize liver function as much as possible given the urgency of the operative procedure. Operations performed under emergency circumstances, especially for hemorrhage, operations immediately following an alcoholic binge, and operations in the acute phase of hepatitis all carry an increased risk. Active hepatocellular inflammation should be allowed to subside. The alcoholic should be allowed to stabilize and gain maximum improvement in liver function, often requiring a period of several weeks. The use of nutritional supplements by mouth if possible but by intravenous alimentation if necessary may aid in this process. Acute bleeding episodes in patients with liver disease should be terminated by nonsurgical means if possible. The use by Nusbaum et al of vasopressin infusion through visceral arteries has made it possible to decrease portal pressure and thus control hemorrhage from esophageal varices in almost every case [7-68]. This experience has been confirmed by others [7-69].

Renal function should be evaluated by measurement of the creatinine clearance, and excess sodium and water removed as much as possible by the use of diuretics. Potassium supplements may be necessary. Coagulation defects must be corrected. Vitamin K should be administered with the hope of improving prothrombin levels. At the time of operation, platelet concentrates and fresh frozen plasma may be required to produce normal coagulation.

INTRAOPERATIVE CARE

Most important is the avoidance of hepatic anoxia. This means that arterial oxygenation and blood-gas profile should be maintained at normal levels at all times. Hypovolemia with vasoconstriction and/or hypotension must be avoided. Excess manipulation of the splanchnic bed may cause reflex vasospasm and decrease in portal blood flow. Renal function must be kept as normal as possible using intraoperative diuresis when necessary. Cardiac function in the hyperdynamic cirrhotic patient must be maintained at an adequate level. Inotropic drugs and digitalis may be necessary. The increased susceptibility to infection which exists in a patient with poor liver function must be kept in mind. Attention must be paid to the maintenance of sterile technique. Prophylactic antibiotics may be indicated under certain circumstances such as operations on the intestinal tract or the placement of vascular prostheses.

POSTOPERATIVE CARE

The necessity for maintenance of all metabolic systems at optimal levels continues throughout the postoperative period. If the operation has been a portosystemic shunt, an increase in liver damage may occur in 72 hours following operation. Maintenance of cardiac function, renal function, and blood-gas normality is vital to survival.

EXCHANGE TRANSFUSION AND LIVER PERFUSION

The liver failure which occurs following massive resection of normal liver tissue is one condition of acute liver failure which clearly warrants the use of exchange transfusion or xenogeneic liver perfusion. In such patients with a small remnant of normal liver remaining, regeneration and improvement in liver function may be expected to occur, and the use of heroic measures to tide the patient over acute hepatic failure is justified. Exchange transfusion also appears to improve survival in cases of fulminant hepatic failure due to hepatitis, especially in the younger age groups [7-70, 7-71].

REFERENCES

7-1.   Mori, K., Quinlan, R., Richter, D., Kaster, R., Tan, B. H., and Gans, H.: Characterization of the acute hepatic failure syndrome associated with the anhepatic state. Surg. Gynec. Obst. 131:919, 1970.

7-2.   Rutherford, R. B., and Hardaway, R. M., III.: Significance of the rate of decrease in fibrinogen level after total hepatectomy in dogs. Ann. Surg. 163:51, 1966.

7-3.   McDermott, W. V., Jr., Greenberger, N. J., Isselbacher, K. J., and Weber, A. L.: Major hepatic resection: Diagnostic techniques and metabolic problems. Surgery 54:56, 1963.

7-4.   Raffucci, F. L., and Ramirez-Schon, G.: Management of tumors of the liver. Surg. Gynec. Obst. 130:371, 1970.

7-5.   Aronsen, K. F., Ericsson, B., and Pihl, B.: Metabolic changes following major hepatic resection. Ann. Surg. 169:102, 1969.

7-6.   Cain, G. D., Mayer, G., and Jones, E. A.: Augmentation of albumin but not fibrinogen synthesis by corticosteroids in patients with hepatocellular disease. J. Clin. Invest. 49:2198, 1970.

7-7.   Rothschild, M. A., Oratz, M., Zimmon, D., Schreiber, S. S., Weiner, I., and Van Caneghem, A.: Albumin synthesis in cirrhotic subjects with ascites studied with carbonate-^{14}C. J. Clin. Invest. 48:344, 1969.

7-8.   Dykes, P. W.: The rates of distribution and catabolism of albumin in normal subjects and in patients with cirrhosis of the liver. Clin. Sci. 34:161, 1968.

7-9.   Allen, H., and Spellberg, M.: Alkaline phosphatase in bile and urine: Excretion in patients with hepatobiliary disease. Arch. Intern. Med. 120:667, 1967.

7-10.   Sebesta, D. G., Bradshaw, F. J., and Prockop, D. J.: Source of the elevated serum alkaline phosphatase activity in biliary obstruction: Studies utilizing isolated liver perfusion. Gastroenterology 47:166, 1964.

7-11.   Almersjo, O., Bengmark, S., Hafstrom, L. O., and Olsson, R.: Enzyme and function changes after extensive liver resection in man. Ann. Surg. 169:111, 1969.

7-12. Nothman, M. M., and Callow, A. D.: Investigations on the origin of amlyase in serum and urine. Gastroenterology 60:82, 1971.

7-13. Grossi, C. E., Rousselot, L. M., and Panke, W. F.: Control of fibrinolysis during portacaval shunts. Study of patients with cirrhosis of the liver. JAMA 187:1005, 1964.

7-14. Walls, W. D., and Losowsky, M. S.: The hemostatic defect of liver disease. Gastroenterology 60:108, 1971.

7-15. Owren, P. A.: The diagnostic and prognostic significance of plasma prothrombin and factor V levels in parenchymatous hepatitis and obstructive jaundice. Scand. J. Clin. Lab. Invest. 1:131, 1949.

7-16. O'Connell, R. A., Grossi, C. E., and Rousselot, L. M.: Role of inhibitors of fibrinolysis in hepatic cirrhosis. Lancet 2:990, 1964.

7-17. Yates, F. E.: Contributions of the liver to steady-state performance and transient responses of the adrenal cortical system. Fed. Proc. 24:733, 1965.

7-18. Magraf, H. W., Moyer, C. A., Ashford, L. E., and Lavalle, L. W.: Adrenocortical function in alcoholics. J. Surg. Res. 7:55, 1967.

7-19. Lauson, H. D.: Antidiuretic hormone. Fed. Proc. 24:731, 1965.

7-20. Koff, R. S., Grady, G. F., Chalmers, T. C., Mosley, J. W., Swartz, B. L., and Boston Inter-Hospital Liver Group: Viral hepatitis in a group of Boston Hospitals. III. Importance of exposure to shellfish in a nonepidemic period. New Engl. J. Med. 276:703, 1967.

7-21. Walsh, J. H., Purcell, R. H., Morrow, A. G., Chanock, R. M., and Schmidt, P. J.: Posttransfusion hepatitis after open-heart operations. JAMA 211:261, 1970.

7-22. Mirick, G. S., Ward, R., and McCollum, R. W.: Modification of posttransfusion hepatitis by gamma globulin. New Engl. J. Med. 273:59, 1965.

7-23. Zimmerman, H. J.: Clinical and laboratory manifestations of hepatotoxicity. Ann. N.Y. Acad. Sci. 104:954, 1963.

7-24. Drill, V. A.: Pharmacology of hepatotoxic agents. Gastroenterology 38:786, 1960.

7-25. Popper, H., and Schaeffner, F.: Drug-induced hepatic injury. Ann. Intern. Med. 51:1230, 1959.

7-26. Ticktin, H. E., and Robinson, M. M.: Effects of some antimicrobial agents on the liver. Ann. N.Y. Acad. Sci. 104:1080, 1963.

7-27. Summerskill, W. H. J., Davidson, C. S., Dible, J. H., Mallory, K., Sherlock, S., Turner, M. D., and Wolfe, S. J.: Cirrhosis of the liver. A study of alcoholic and nonalcoholic patients in Boston and London. New Engl. J. Med. 262:1, 1960.

7-28. Garceau, A. J., and Boston Inter-Hospital Liver Group: The natural history of cirrhosis. II. The influence of alcohol and prior hepatitis on pathology and prognosis. New Engl. J. Med. 271:1174, 1964.

7-29.   Mendelson, J. H.: Biologic concomitants of alcoholism. New Engl. J. Med. 283:24, 1970.

7-30.   Owens, A. H., Jr., and Marshall, E. K., Jr.: The metabolism of ethyl alcohol in the rat. J. Pharmacol. Exp. Ther. 115:360, 1955.

7-31.   Smith, M. E., and Newman, H. W.: The rate of ethanol metabolism in fed and fasting animals. J. Biol. Chem. 234:1544, 1959.

7-32.   Hayes, M. A., Hodgson, P. E., and Coller, F. A.: The use of testosterone in preventing postoperative liver dysfunction in the poor risk surgical patient. Ann. Surg. 136:643, 1952.

7-33.   Mendelson, J. H.: Biologic concomitants of alcoholism (second of two parts). New Engl. J. Med. 283:71, 1970.

7-34.   Price, H. L., Deutsch, S., Marshall, B. E., Stephen, G. W., Behar, M. G., and Neufeld, G. R.: Hemodynamic and metabolic effects of hemorrhage in man, with particular reference to the splanchnic circulation. Circ. Res. 18:469, 1966.

7-35.   Ellenberg, M., and Osserman, K. E.: The role of shock in the production of central liver cell necrosis. Am. J. Med. 11:170, 1951.

7-36.   Vanecko, R. M., Szanto, P. B., and Shoemaker, W. C.: Microcirculatory changes in primate liver during shock. Surg. Gynec. Obst. 129:995, 1969.

7-37.   DePalma, R. G., Levey, S., and Holden, W. D.: Ultrastructure and oxidative phosphorylation of liver mitochondria in experimental hemorrhagic shock. J. Trauma 10:122, 1970.

7-38.   Monafo, W. W., Jr., Ternberg, J. L., and Kempson, R.: Accidental ligation of the hepatic artery. Arch. Surg. 92:643, 1966.

7-39.   Farkouh, E. F., Daniel, A. M., Beaudoin, J.-G., and MacLean, L. D.: Predictive value of liver biochemistry in acute hepatic ischemia. Surg. Gynec. Obst. 132:832, 1971.

7-40.   Abouna, G. M., Aldrete, J. A., and Starzl, T. E.: Changes in serum potassium and pH during clinical and experimental liver transplantation. Surgery 69:419, 1971.

7-41.   Alican, F., Cayirli, M., and Keith, V.: Fibrinolytic activity following experimental procedures on the liver. Arch. Surg. 101:590, 1970.

7-42.   Rangel, D. M., Dinbar, A., Stevens, G. H., Cooper, R., and Fonkalsrud, E. W.: The hepatic response to endotoxin shock: Hemodynamic and enzymatic observations. J. Surg. Res. 10:181, 1970.

7-43.   Schumer, W., Das Gupta, T. K., Moss, G. S., and Nyhus, L. M.: Effect of endotoxemia on liver cell mitochondria in man. Ann. Surg. 171:875, 1970.

7-44.   Rangel, D. M., Byfield, J. E., Adomian, G. E., Stevens, G. H., and Fonkalsrud, E. W.: Hepatic ultrastructural response to endotoxin shock. Surgery 68:503, 1970.

7-45.   Fisher, E. R., and McCloy, D.: Hepatic lesions of acute hemorrhagic pancreatitis. Their nature and pathogenesis. Surgery 37:213, 1955.

7-46.   Scott, R., Jr., Howard, J. M., and Olney, J. M., Jr.: Hepatic function of the battle casualty; the systemic response to injury. Surg. Gynec. Obst. 102:209, 1956.

7-47. Ravdin, I. S., and Vars, H. M.: Further studies on factors influencing liver injury and liver repair. Ann. Surg. 132:362, 1950.

7-48. Harrah, J. D., Holmes, E. C., Paulson, D. F., and Ketcham, A. S.: Serum enzyme alterations after extensive surgical procedures. Ann. Surg. 169:300, 1969.

7-49. Strasbert, S. M., and Silver, M. D.: Postoperative hepatogenic jaundice. Surg. Gynec. Obst. 132:81, 1971.

7-50. Nunes, G., Blaisdell, W., and Margaretten, W.: Mechanism of hepatic dysfunction following shock and trauma. Arch. Surg. 100:546, 1970.

7-51. Kantrowitz, P. A., Jones, W. A., Greenberger, N. J., and Isselbacher, K. J.: Severe postoperative hyperbilirubinemia simulating obstructive jaundice. New Engl. J. Med. 276:591, 1967.

7-52. Siegel, J. H., Greenspan, M., Cohn, J. D., and DelGuercio, L. R. M.: The prognostic implications of altered physiology in operations for portal hypertension. Surg. Gynec. Obst. 126:249, 1968.

7-53. Siegel, J. H., and Williams, J. B.: A computer based index for the prediction of operative survival in patients with cirrhosis and portal hypertension. Ann. Surg. 169:191, 1969.

7-54. DelGuercio, L. R. M., Commaraswamy, R. P., Feins, N. R., Wollman, S. B., and State, D.: Pulmonary arteriovenous admixture and the hyperdynamic cardiovascular state in surgery for portal hypertension. Surgery 56:57, 1964.

7-55. Murray, J. F., Dawson, A. M., and Sherlock, S.: Circulatory changes in chronic liver disease. Am. J. Med. 24:358, 1958.

7-56. Mashford, M. L., Mahon, W. A., and Chalmers, T. C.: Studies of the cardiovascular system in the hypotension of liver failure. New Engl. J. Med. 267:1071, 1962.

7-57. Chidsey, C. A., Kaiser, G. A., Sonnenblick, E. H., Spann, J. F., and Braunwald, E.: Cardiac norepinephrine stores in experimental heart failure in the dog. J. Clin. Invest. 43:2386, 1964.

7-58. Koppel, M. H., Coburn, J. W., Mims, M. M., Goldstein, H., Boyle, J. D., and Rubini, M. E.: Transplantation of cadaveric kidneys from patients with hepatorenal syndrome. Evidence for the functional nature of renal failure in advanced liver disease. New Engl. J. Med. 280:1367, 1969.

7-59. Baldus, W. P., Summerskill, W. H. J., Hunt, J. C., and Maher, F. T.: Renal circulation in cirrhosis: Observations based on catheterization of the renal vein. J. Clin. Invest. 43:1090, 1964.

7-60. Epstein, M., Berk, D. P., Hollenberg, N. K., Adams, D. F., Chalmers, T. C., Abrams, H. L., and Merrill, J. P.: Renal failure in the patient with cirrhosis: The role of active vasoconstriction. Am. J. Med. 49:175, 1970.

7-61. Mullane, J. F., and Gliedman, M. L.: Elevation of the pressure in the abdominal inferior vena cava as a cause of a hepatorenal syndrome in cirrhosis. Surgery 59:1135, 1966.

7-62: Wakui, K., DeCosse, J. J., Vanamee, P., and Lawrence, W., Jr.: Effect of increased intraperitoneal pressure on renal function. Surg. Forum 13:387, 1962.

7-63. Tristani, F. E., and Cohn, J. N.: Systemic and renal hemodynamics in oliguric hepatic failure: Effect of volume expansion. J. Clin. Invest. 46:1894, 1967.

7-64. Norman, J. C., Saravis, C. A., Brown, M. E., and McDermott, W. V., Jr.: Immunochemical observations in clinical heterologous (xenogeneic) liver perfusion. Surgery 60:179, 1966.

7-65. Linton, R. R.: The selection of patients for portacaval shunt with a summary of the results in 61 cases. Ann. Surg. 134:433, 1951.

7-66. McDermott, W. V., Jr., Palazzi, H., Nardi, G. L., and Mondet, A.: Elective portal systemic shunt. An analysis of 237 cases. New Engl. J. Med. 264:419, 1961.

7-67. Child, C. G., III: The portal circulation. New Engl. J. Med. 252:837, 1955.

7-68. Nusbaum, M., Baum, S., Kuroda, K., and Blakemore, W. S.: Control of portal hypertension by selective mesenteric arterial drug infusion. Arch. Surg. 97:1005, 1968.

7-69. Stahl, W. M.: Evaluation of cirrhotic patient for surgery. N.Y. State J. Med. 71:570, 1971.

7-70. Trey, C.: The fulminant hepatic failure surveillance study. Brief review of the effects of presumed etiology and age of survival. Canad. Med. Ass. J. 106:525, 1972.

7-71. Klebanoff, G., Hollander, D., Cosimi, A. B., Stanford, W., and Kemmerer, W. T.: Asanguineous hypothermic total body perfusion (TBW) in the treatment of stage IV hepatic coma. J. Surg. Res. 12:1, 1972.

8

ENDOCRINES

PANCREAS

The pancreas contributes to the maintenance of normal body function by exocrine secretion into the gastrointestinal tract, and by endocrine secretion of hormones, the most important of which is insulin.

Insulin

Insulin is a hormone of approximately 6000 molecular weight, consisting of two polypeptide chains. It is manufactured in the beta cells, collected within the cell in granules, and discharged into the blood stream as a response to elevation of the blood glucose. Insulin acts to promote the transfer of glucose across certain cell membranes. Cells which require insulin for glucose transport are those of skeletal and cardiac muscle, fibroblasts, mammary tissue, anterior pituitary, the lens of the eye, and the aorta. Other tissues do not require insulin for the transfer of glucose. These tissues include nerve tissue, erthyrocytes, intestinal mucosal cells, kidney tubules, and liver cells [8-1].

Effects of Insulin Lack

Lack of sufficient insulin decreases glucose entry into insulin sensitive cells. This together with gluconeogenesis leads to hyperglycemia and glycosuria. Osmotic diuresis results with subsequent dehydration.

205

Insulin lack also causes fat to be mobilized as free fatty acid and as triglyceride. Ketonemia results because of accumulation of acetoacetic acid and betahydroxybuteric acid. With fall in glucose metabolism, protein catabolism occurs, especially in muscle. Protein potassium is liberated and lost in the urine. Acidosis is increased. Progressive dehydration, loss of sodium and potassium, and increase in acid products lead to coma and eventual death [8-2].

Diabetes Mellitus

Diabetes mellitus is a genetically determined disease. In this disease an abnormality of the interrelationship between insulin, glucagon, and carbohydrate metabolism occurs which exposes the patient to the effects of insulin deprivation unless appropriate diet and/or insulin therapy is used.

The development of the radioimmunoassay technique for the measurement of circulating insulin has improved the understanding of the diabetic state [8-3]. In diabetic patients insulin secretion in response to the administration of glucose is delayed and insulin levels remain high for a longer time than in the normal individual [8-4]. Insulin sensitivity appears to be impaired [8-5] and insulin levels actually are low compared to the level of glucose. Hypovolemia and potassium deficits seem to further decrease carbohydrate tolerance in these patients [8-6].

VASCULAR LESIONS

Alterations of the basement membrane of capillaries has been found in overtly diabetic patients and in a high percentage of genetically prediabetic individuals [8-7]. This microangiopathy appears to be an early lesion in the diabetic syndrome and seems independent of the carbohydrate derangements. Although this lesion is still poorly understood, it is of vital importance since vascular complications constitute the major causes of death in patients with treated diabetes mellitus. Such vascular complications are manifested by the development of atherosclerosis of large and medium-sized vessels and of the smaller arterioles. Peripheral effects are seen most often in the legs. Centrally, renal damage due to thickening of the basement membrane as described by Kimmelstiel and Wilson [8-8] (nodular glomerulosclerosis) or by Fahr [8-9] (diffuse glomerulosclerosis) may lead to severe renal damage with renal failure. Microangiopathy produces especially severe changes in the retinal vessels. Diabetic retinopathy very often progresses to complete blindness [8-10].

NEUROPATHY

Interference with normal functioning of nerves occurs often in diabetes, apparently from the disturbance in metabolism of nerve cells [8-11]. The spotty and focal nature of the lesion suggests that it is not due directly to the diabetic microangiopathy. Peripheral nerves, especially in the lower extremities, may be involved with the production of pain and paresthesias. Muscular weakness and absence of knee and ankle jerks may occur. In addition, neuropathy can occur in the gastrointestinal tract with delay in gastric emptying, intermittent diarrhea, and alteration in small-bowel function. Loss of activity of the detrusor muscle of the bladder may occur causing a picture mimicking "cord bladder." Involvement of the autonomic nervous system may simulate sympathectomy with the occurrence of postural hypotension, vasomotor instability, tachycardia, and dependent edema [8-12].

SUSCEPTIBILITY TO INFECTION

The patient with diabetes has decreased resistance to infection. The exact mechanism producing this lack of resistance is not known. Impaired mobilization of leukocytes to infected sites has been suggested [8-13]. An increase in serum osmolarity with interference with capillary flow is also a possible explanation [8-14]. Acidosis has been shown to interfere with cellular defense against infection [8-15]. Basement membrane alterations due to the microangiopathy itself may be involved.

PREOPERATIVE MANAGEMENT

Patients suffering from diabetes mellitus require special care when operation is needed. The stress of trauma, sepsis, and anxiety, and the alterations produced by anesthesia, fluid shifts, and nutritional changes may exacerbate the diabetic state. The preoperative evaluation should include a careful documentation of the history of the patient with regard to his diabetes. A search for diabetes mellitus by history and physical examination is important in any patient, and in one series more than 20 per cent of a large group of patients were found to be diabetic only on the occasion of their admission to a hospital for operation [8-16]. In such patients the presence of obesity is common and the complications due to atherosclerosis, neuropathy, retinopathy, and nephropathy must be kept in mind. Evaluation of the function of these vital systems must be made prior to any contemplated operation.

Emergency Operations.   Emergency operations are required more often in diabetics than in normal individuals and the preoperative preparation may have to be carried out over a short period of time. In the presence of sepsis, delay in operation may be dangerous to the patient, since insulin resistance and metabolic decompensation will respond only after the infection is controlled.

INTRAOPERATIVE MANAGEMENT

The management of the patient during his operative procedure is aimed at preventing an excessive rise or fall in the blood sugar, preventing excessive urinary glucose losses and acidosis. If this can be done, the predisposition to infection is reduced and nutritional failure due to glycogenolysis is avoided. Anesthetic agents usually have little effect on the blood sugar.

A satisfactory management schedule should include determination of the fasting blood sugar level prior to operation. Administration of needed glucose is achieved by giving a solution of 5 per cent dextrose in water intravenously. Regular insulin should be given subcutaneously using a sliding scale of 15, 10, 5, and 0 units, based on a urine test every four hours. In some cases the morning administration of 10 to 20 units of long-acting insulin with supplemental regular insulin is a satisfactory procedure [8-17]. A blood-sugar level should be drawn on the afternoon following operation and more often if indicated.

POSTOPERATIVE CARE

The postoperative course is similar to that in the nondiabetic patient. Glucose is given by vein until the patient can take food by mouth. The administration of regular insulin by four-hour urine test is a satisfactory method to use until the patient's regular maintenance schedule can be resumed. The increased incidence of vascular complications including myocardial infarction, and of septic complications in the urinary tract, lungs, and elsewhere must be kept in mind.

Glucagon

Glucagon, a hormone secreted by the alpha cells, produces hyperglycemia and has an inotropic effect on cardiac action [8-18]. In its action it opposes the effect of insulin. Together these two hormones control the movement of glucose and certain amino acids in and out of body cells in accordance with the need for energy and the availability of fuel substances [8-19]. The insulin-glucagon ratio thus appears to be more important than the actual insulin level in fine regulation of glucose metabolism. Infusion of glucose or of lipid as triglyceride stimulates beta-cell secretion with a rise in insulin levels, and inhibits alpha-cell secretion with a fall in glucagon. Infusion of amino acids on the other hand causes a rise in both hormones. Insulin aids in incorporation of amino acid into protein, a process which requires glucose entry into cells [8-20]. Glucagon prevents a fall in blood glucose level by releasing glucose from the liver [8-21]. Glucagon secretion appears to be elevated in the diabetic individual, both in the fasting state [8-22], after a protein meal [8-23], and after administration of carbohydrate [8-23].

The administration of exogenous glucagon is used mainly for its cardiac stimulatory effects. The concomitant hyperglycemic effect must be kept in mind.

Other Hormones

Metabolic disturbances resulting from secretion of other substances by pancreatic cells have been recognized only in those patients where tumors of specific cell types release abnormally large amounts of hormone into the circulation. The production of a gastrinlike substance stimulates massive hypersecretion of acid by the fundic cells of the stomach, resulting in the fulminating ulcer diathesis of the Zollinger-Ellison syndrome. Production of a secretinlike hormone causes intestinal hypersecretion and diarrhea.

THYROID

Thyroxin

The biologic role of thyroxin is not precisely known. This hormone, however, seems to act predominantly on the respiratory enzyme systems of mitochondria. An appropriate level of hormone appears to be necessary for the adequate production of messenger RNA, probably via action on cyclic AMP. The synthesis of proteins, including mitochondrial enzymes, depends upon the presence of proper amounts of thyroid hormone. Reaction to catecholamines also seems to depend on the presence of thyroxin, which especially affects the receptivity of beta receptors.

Hyperthyroidism

Hyperthyroidism is due to the presence of an increased amount of active hormone. All tissue cells appear to be effected, but measured changes are especially severe in the liver and in muscle. Oxygen consumption is increased as is heat production. Activity of the mitochondrial enzyme system is increased and the mitochondria actually increase in size. However, the efficiency of ATP production is decreased and greater oxygen consumption is required per molecule of ATP. Sensitivity to catecholamines appears to be increased.

GENERAL CLINICAL PICTURE

These general reactions explain the clinical picture seen in hyperthyroidism. The patient is restless, irritable, and hyperkinetic with an increased basal metabolic rate. Nutritional imbalance may be present with a special decrease in lean muscle tissue [8-24]. The function of skeletal muscle is altered. The development of force by muscle contraction is normal, but the duration of the active contractile state is shortened. Weakness may therefore be produced by lack of fusion of the contracting muscle fibers [8-25].

CARDIOVASCULAR EFFECTS

Cardiovascular changes are those of an increase in cardiac output with a hyperdynamic circulation [8-26]. Cardiac contraction seems to be somewhat less efficient than normal, and the workload of the heart seems to be increased, since cardiac output levels are abnormally high for a given oxygen consumption [8-27]. This hyperdynamic state of the heart is caused both by an increase in rate and an increase in stroke volume, perhaps due to sensitization to the effects of catecholamines [8-28].

RESPIRATORY EFFECTS

Alterations in ventilatory capacity are also seen with hyperthyroidism [8-27]. In such patients an increase in minute ventilation is necessary because of the increased oxygen consumption. However, minute ventilation is excessive even in relation to this increased oxygen uptake. Studies have shown a reduction in vital capacity and in expiratory reserve volume with an increase in respiratory frequency. This change has been ascribed to weakness of the respiratory muscles due to the direct muscle effect of thyroid hormone.

INTESTINAL EFFECTS

The effects on the intestinal tract consist of increased appetite and hypermotility with rapid glucose absorption.

RESPONSE TO STRESS

Alteration in the basic energy-production system of body cells due to hyperthyroidism interferes with the normal response to stress and trauma. Appropriate increases in cardiovascular activity in response to injury may not be possible. Protein synthesis is impaired, wound healing suffers, and susceptibility to infection is increased.

THYROID STORM

The danger of uncontrollable hyperthyroidism or thyrotoxic storm is always present. This crisis is usually of abrupt onset and may be precipitated by stress of any sort. The characteristic clinical picture includes hyperpyrexia, sometimes in excess of 106°F, and excess stimulation of the cardiovascular system with the production of congestive failure and pulmonary edema. Central nervous system symptoms include tremor, restlessness, confusion, and psychosis, progressing to apathy and coma. Abnormalities of liver function occur with hepatomegaly and jaundice. Hyperactivity of the gastrointestinal tract may be a significant part of the clinical picture with diarrhea, abdominal pain, and nausea, and vomiting. The clinical picture may occasionally suggest an acute abdominal emergency [8-29].

Hypothyroidism

Hypothyroidism due to insufficient production of thyroid hormone produces the reverse effect on the organism. Oxygen consumption and energy production by mitochondria are decreased, although efficiency of phosphorylation is normal. Oxygen uptake is low with a decrease in the basal metabolic rate. Production of protein, especially enzyme protein, is decreased. Hypercholesterolemia occurs because the metabolism of cholesterol is decreased to a greater degree than the decrease in cholesterol production. Skeletal-muscle contraction is affected with a fall in the maximum force produced [8-25]. The circulation becomes hypodynamic with a decrease in cardiac output, blood pressure, and an increase in circulation time. Cardiac contractility is impaired. Gastrointestinal function is decreased with loss of appetite and poor absorption of glucose. Susceptibility to infection is increased, perhaps due to changes in the immune mechanism or to decrease in phagocytic activity of leukocytes.

Effect of Trauma on Thyroid Function

It has been suggested that surgery and trauma produce changes in thyroid function which contribute to the total endocrine disturbance occurring after injury [8-30]. Increased utilization of thyroid hormone by peripheral tissues has been suggested, since radioactive iodine uptake by the thyroid is increased while blood levels of hormone remain normal [8-31]. Activation of change in thyroid function would appear to operate at a deeper level than activation of change in adrenal cortical response, because exposure to cold activates the latter but not the former [8-32]. The interrelationships between corticosteroid and thyroid hormones are complex and the normal adrenal response to stress may counteract any tendency toward rise in thyroid hormone production [8-33].

Preoperative Evaluation

The poor response of either the hyper- or hypothyroid patient to the trauma of operation makes it vitally important to assess the level of thyroid function of every preoperative patient. Ordinarily the diagnosis is made on clinical grounds alone as most patients show the classic picture of hyper- or hypothyroidism. Hyperthyroidism, however, may be masked, especially in the older individual. In such patients hyperdynamic cardiac action may be the only sign and the presence of cardiac arrhythmia should lead one to suspect possible occult hyperthyroidism.

TESTS FOR THYROID FUNCTION

Presently accepted tests for thyroid function include the measurement of serum thyroxin and tri-iodothyronine, T-3 resin uptake, measurement of the protein bound iodine, and assessment of the radioactive iodine uptake of the thyroid gland. In a small percentage of cases, hyperthyroidism may be due to elevation of the serum tri-iodothyronine level alone. In such patients this value will be elevated while all other tests may be normal [8-34].

Preoperative Preparation

Control of hyperthyroidism by the administration of iodine, or anti-thyroid drugs such as propylthiouracil or Tapazole (methimazole), and in acute cases the use of beta blockers, namely propranalol, is of utmost importance prior to operation if time permits. In the emergency situation the use of iodine, beta blockade, and sympatholytic drugs may be entertained. For patients with hypothyroidism, the return of body metabolism to normal by administration of crude thyroid or purified hormone is essential before operation is performed.

PARATHYROID

The importance of calcium homeostasis in the maintenance of normal neuromuscular excitability has been recognized for some time. Central to the maintenance of normal serum calcium levels is appropriate secretion of hormone by the parathyroid glands.

Control of Parathyroid Hormone Secretion

Secretion of parathyroid hormone is regulated by the level of ionized serum calcium [8-35, 8-36]. Acid-base balance also plays an important part in regulating the release of parathyroid hormone because of its effect on ionized calcium. When alkalosis occurs, ionized calcium is decreased and parathyroid hormone stimulated [8-37]. The increase in parathyroid hormone production in chronic renal disease apparently is caused by the effect of phosphate retention with hyperphosphatemia and secondary hypocalcemia [8-38].

Action of Parathyroid Hormone

Parathyroid hormone acts through mobilizing calcium from bone and by causing an increase in urinary phosphate excretion [8-39]. Both of these actions may be mediated through the formation of cyclic 3,5-AMP at the cell membrane [8-40, 8-41].

Hyperparathyroidism

Hyperfunction of the parathyroid gland is most frequently encountered as primary hyperparathyroidism due to tumor or hyperplasia of the parathyroid gland [8-42, 8-43].

DIAGNOSIS

The most valuable diagnostic measurement in such cases is elevation of the serum calcium. Ordinarily, approximately 40 per cent of plasma calcium is bound to protein and the amount so bound depends on the level of calcium and of protein, predominantly albumin. Evaluation of the total calcium level must be made with due regard for the level of the circulating albumin in the patient, since symptoms apparently depend on elevation of the ionized fraction [8-44]. Other tests which may be used are measurement of the serum phosphorus which is usually increased, and measurement of the tubular resorption of phosphate which is usually below 80 per cent. Since the development of a radioimmunoassay of plasma levels of parathyroid hormone, the diagnosis has become more precise [8-45]. The autonomous nature of a parathyroid hypersecreting tumor can be determined by failure of parathyroid hormone secretion to be altered by calcium infusion.

CLINICAL PICTURE

Hyperparathyroidism, with mild degrees of hypercalcemia, can exist with no symptoms whatsoever. The increased use of screening biochemical techniques has shown a hitherto unsuspected group of patients harboring parathyroid adenoma without symptoms [8-46]. Mild to moderate degrees of hypercalcemia are often associated with relatively nonspecific symptoms such as constipation, dyspepsia, lassitude, easy fatigue, and polyuria. Renal stones are formed in a high percentage of patients due to the increase in calcium in the urine. Any patient with renal calculi should therefore be screened for the presence of hyperparathyroidism. The incidence of peptic ulcer appears to be increased, and gastric hypersecretion has been implicated [8-47, 8-48]. Pancreatitis also occurs with increased frequency [8-42]. Increased levels of glucagon have been measured, and pancreatic islet cell hyperplasia has been reported [8-49].

PARATHYROID STORM

Severe and fatal disturbances may be caused by rapid rise in the serum calcium [8-50]. This condition has been called *hypercalcemic crisis* or *parathyroid storm* and usually presents with weakness, intractable nausea and vomiting, dehydration, and coma. The electrocardiogram shows shortening of the ST intervals, and kidney function is decreased with a fall in the GFR, interference with concentration, loss of potassium, and increase in calcium excretion. Urgent treatment is needed to prevent a fatal outcome. The use of phosphate infusion [8-51] and sodium sulfate infusion has been suggested [8-52]. The marked effect of ethacrynic acid diuresis in enhancing calcium excretion in the urine has been used for the treatment of hypercalcemia. Rapid reduction of serum calcium is possible due to the excretion of large amounts of calcium. The use of diuresis with this agent should be considered as the primary treatment for acute symptomatic hypercalcemia [8-53].

Other Causes of Hypercalcemia

Hypercalcemia may occur due to conditions other than hyperparathyroidism. Tumors of other tissues, namely lung, adrenal, and parotid, have been shown to produce a parathyroid hormonelike material, in some cases identical with parathyroid hormone on radioimmunoassay [8-54, 8-55]. Occasionally hypercalcemia has been present in patients suffering from myeloma, lymphoma, sarcoid, vitamin D intoxication, hyperthyroidism, and milk-alkali syndrome [8-56]. In addition, serious hypercalcemia may occur in the course of therapy of osseous metastases with steroids [8-57].

Hypoparathyroidism

Hypoparathyroidism is most commonly encountered following inadvertent damage to or removal of the parathyroid glands during thyroid operations. Hypocalcemia develops, stabilizing at approximately 6 mg %, where it remains in equilibrium with the labile calcium of the skeleton [8-58]. Neuromuscular irritability is present with tetany and a positive Chvostek sign. Hypocalcemic convulsions and death may occur. In such patients parathyroid hormone cannot be detected in the serum [8-38].

Treatment of such primary hypoparathyroidism involves the administration of calcium and large doses of vitamin D. Vitamin D appears to raise serum calcium concentrations by its effect on enhancing calcium absorption, mobilizing bone calcium, and increasing urinary phosphate excretion. The mechanism of these effects is not well understood. The difficulty of precise control of hypoparathyroidism by vitamin D has been pointed out [8-59]. Most patients require at least 1.25 mg per day for therapeutic effect, but over 2.50 mg per day may produce hypercalcemia. In addition to this narrow margin between therapeutic and toxic dosage, the response of a given patient may vary. Increase in serum calcium may occur weeks after discontinuance of therapy. Serum levels must be measured frequently.

PSEUDOHYPOPARATHYROIDISM: THYROCALCITONIN

Pseudohypoparathyroidism may present with hypocalcemia but with increased quantities of parathyroid hormone in the circulation [8-38]. In two such patients the thyroid gland has shown an increased concentration of thyrocalcitonin, a thyroid hormone which produces hypocalcemia and hypophosphatemia [8-60]. This hormone is a small polypeptide produced in the parafollicular cell of the thyroid, a cell which appears to be derived from the ultimobranchial tissue [8-61]. The action of thyrocalcitonin appears to be directly on bone to inhibit calcium mobilization [8-62]. Although it seems to have an important effect in lower animals, its importance in man has yet to be determined, unless it can be implicated in pseudohypoparathyroidism.

LATE EFFECTS OF HYPOCALCEMIA

The importance of careful follow-up over the long term in cases of hypoparathyroidism has been stressed [8-63]. Late, irreversible sequelae, including cataract, convulsive disorders, and mental deterioration can occur if hypocalcemia persists.

ADRENAL CORTEX

The regulatory functions of the adrenal cortical hormones are exceedingly complex due to the large number of compounds synthesized and the multiplicity of their effects. In general, adrenal cortical hormones can be grouped into the sex steroids, androgens and estrogens; the glucocorticoids, of which cortisol is a prototype; and the mineralocorticoids, represented by aldosterone.

Regulation of Glucocorticoid Secretion

Cortisol synthesis by the zona fasciculata of the adrenal cortex is stimulated by adrenocorticotrophic hormone (ACTH) [8-64]. Discharge of this anterior pituitary hormone is in turn regulated by the level of corticotrophin-releasing factor, a neurohormone elaborated by the hypothalamus. Cortisol concentrations in the blood exert a negative feedback control over this factor, and thus over ACTH release. ACTH and cortisol secretion shows a cyclic variation with lowest levels near midnight and highest levels at 8 or 9 A.M. Basal cortisol secretion varies from 10 to 28 mg/24 hr. Cortisol is metabolized by the liver and the metabolic products excreted in the urine. Approximately 50 per cent of these metabolites retain the dihydroxyacetone side chain at carbon 17 and are identified in the urine as 17-hydroxycorticosteroids.

Glucocorticoid Insufficiency

Adrenal cortical insufficiency may be spontaneous or postsurgical, or may be produced by depression of normal responsiveness of the adrenal cortex due to the administration of exogenous hormone [8-65, 8-66].

CARDIOVASCULAR EFFECTS

The most common sign of adrenal insufficiency is unexplained hypotension [8-67]. The main cause of instability of the circulation in the absence of adequate glucocorticoid levels appears to be functional impairment of the myocardium [8-68]. Both the rate of rise of ventricular pressure (dp/dt) and the maximum pressure achieved are depressed in adrenal insufficiency [8-69]. Hypotension itself and hypovolemia normally stimulate secretion of 17-hydroxycorticoids [8-70]. Absence of this increased secretion results in a poor response to hemorrhage and death of the experimental animal [8-71]. Normal production of glucocorticoids appears to be necessary to allow capillary refill after hemorrhage [8-71], and to mobilize cell water to refill the extracellular space [8-72].

RESISTANCE TO INFECTION

An appropriate level of 17-hydroxycorticosteroids is needed to maintain normal resistance to infection. Susceptibility to invasive sepsis increases with either hypo- or hypersecretion of these hormones [8-73].

GLUCOSE METABOLISM

Appropriate levels of glucocorticoids are needed to maintain blood glucose and tissue glycogen levels in the normal range and to allow mobilization of muscle protein for gluconeogenesis during fasting or response to injury [8-74]. These actions apparently result from the effect of these steroids in increasing messenger RNA with the production of a protein that inhibits glucose transport in certain peripheral tissues. Catabolism thus is induced in lymphoid tissue, skin, and adipose tissue. Protein synthesis, and the level of metabolic enzymes in the liver are concomitantly increased [8-75].

Glucocorticoid Excess

ADRENOGENITAL SYNDROME

Congenital adrenocortical hyperplasia has been recognized as an inborn error of metabolism [8-76]. Defective biosynthesis of cortisol allows the accumulation of abnormal steroid metabolites, many with androgenic activity. Virilization is the most common clinical manifestation, usually apparent in the female at birth, and noted in the male later in infancy or childhood. Medical therapy with appropriate steroids is essential to avoid serious complications.

CUSHING'S SYNDROME

In 1912 Harvey Cushing described patients presenting with hypertension, weight gain, hirsutism, moon facies, truncal obesity, striae, and impaired carbohydrate metabolism [8-77]. His patients suffered from basophilic adenoma of the pituitary, but the effects were produced by the increased adrenocorticoid secretion [8-78]. At least four different entities are now recognized as causing this syndrome [8-79]. Most common is dysfunction of the hypothalamic-pituitary axis with resulting adrenal hyperfunction and hyperplasia. Some of these patients may show an obvious pituitary tumor although most do not. Second are the autonomous hyperfunctioning adrenal cortical adenomas, and third, the cortical carcinomas. Lastly, there are extra-adrenal carcinomas which produce an ACTH-like substance, resulting in adrenal hyperplasia. These are most frequently oat-cell carcinomas of the lung and thymic tumors.

The diurnal variation in excretion of 17-hydroxycorticoids is abolished in patients with Cushing's syndrome, and elevated levels of cortisol are found in the serum. Those patients with adrenocortical hyperfunction may be differentiated from those with autonomous tumor by the dexamethasone suppression test. In the former group the hypersecretion is suppressed over 60 per cent by the administration of 2 mg of dexamethasone per day for three days, and then 8 mg per day for three days. Therapy is directed toward the primary cause if possible [8-80].

Regulation of Mineralocorticoid Secretion

Regulation of aldosterone secretion normally depends upon volume sensing by the kidney [8-81]. The exact stimulus is unknown but may be related to renal interstitial pressure and/or tubular sodium concentration. Juxtaglomerular cells release renin into the circulation. Renin is converted to angiotensin I and then to angiotensin II. This latter substance stimulates the zona glomerulosa of the adrenal to secrete aldosterone [8-82]. The effect of aldosterone secretion is to retain sodium and water which restores extracellular volume, and thus complete a closed-loop feedback system. In addition, aldosterone secretion is stimulated by elevated potassium levels in the plasma [8-81].

Mineralocorticoid Insufficiency

The mineralocorticoids, especially aldosterone, have primary action on regulation of the extracellular fluid volume through regulation of sodium resorption in the distal renal tubule. Decrease in the secretion of aldosterone below optimal levels results in loss of sodium, decrease in extracellular fluid volume, and hyponatremia. These abnormalities contribute to circulatory instability.

Mineralocorticoid Excess

Hyperaldosteronism due to tumor or hyperplasia of the zona glomerulosa cell results in sodium retention, edema, hypertension, and hypokalemia. Hypertension is usually the predominant clinical finding [8-82, 8-83]. This primary aldosteronism may be differentiated from the aldosteronism of renal hypertension by the finding of decreased plasma renin levels in the former, and increased plasma renin levels in the latter [8-84].

Cortical Response to Stress

Participation of the adrenal cortex in the normal response to injury was suggested by early workers in the field of stress and trauma

[8-85, 8-86, 8-87]. The rapid and massive increase in urinary excretion of 17-hydroxycorticoids was first documented by Moore and coworkers in patients following trauma and operation [8-88, 8-89]. Direct measurement of the hormone content of adrenal venous effluent corroborated the increase in hormone secretion produced by operation [8-90]. Release of cortical hormone under these conditions is stimulated by ACTH secreted by the pituitary [8-91]. ACTH is stimulated by increase in levels of adrenocorticotrophin-releasing hormone [8-92].

The adrenal cortex must respond with increased secretion of steroids to permit the individual to survive the stress of shock and trauma [8-93]. Failure to increase secretion to an adequate level under these circumstances may precipitate acute adrenal insufficiency in a patient who has not demonstrated insufficiency under normal conditions. This situation may be due to primary adrenal insufficiency, but at present is more often the result of chronic suppression of adrenal function from exogenous corticoid administration. A period of administration lasting one to two weeks at any time within several years can suppress cortical cells to the point where a normal stress response is not possible.

Tests for Adequacy of Adrenal Cortical Function

It is important to test for responsiveness of the adrenal cortex if functional insufficiency is suspected preoperatively. With the development of methodology for the measurement of 17-hydroxycorticosteroids in blood, functional testing of adrenal cortical secretion has become possible [8-94]. Appropriate tests which may be used are the plasma ACTH test and the urinary ACTH test. In the plasma ACTH test a normal response is a rise of greater than 10 mcg/100 ml of plasma, 30 min after the administration of 25 units of ACTH [8-95]. The urinary ACTH test involves collection of a 24-hr control urine and the subsequent collection of a 24-hr urine specimen following the intravenous administration of 25 units of ACTH. A three- to fivefold increase in urinary 17-hydroxysteroids is the normal response [8-95].

Hypoglycemia stimulates adrenal cortical secretion, and this function has been used as a method of assessing the reactivity of the adrenal cortex [8-96]. The increase in cortisol levels appears to be related to the magnitude of fall in blood sugar. Plasma corticosteroid levels also respond to the injection of vasopressin [8-97]. In this test an increase in cortisol levels of greater than 5 mcg/100 ml should occur within 60 min of the injection of 10 pressor units of lysine-B-vasopressin.

Aldosterone insufficiency can usually be detected by a decrease in serum sodium and evidence of decrease in extracellular fluid volume. Abnormally elevated urinary sodium in the presence of hyponatremia is also indicative of inadequate mineralocorticoid secretion, if renal function is normal [8-98].

ADRENAL MEDULLA

The catecholamines, epinephrine and norepinephrine, are synthesized and secreted by the adrenal medulla. In addition to this secretion, catecholamines are synthesized in the brain, in sympathetic nerve endings, and in chromaffin cells of peripheral tissues. Circulating epinephrine is derived almost entirely from the adrenal medulla, while the norepinephrine in the circulation is derived to a considerable degree from sympathetic nerve endings.

Catecholamines delivered to the circulation have a half-life of approximately 10–30 sec [8-99]. Delivery of catecholamine to a target organ therefore depends on the fractional perfusion of that organ in the one minute subsequent to the secretion of hormone into the blood stream. In most organs catecholamine is taken up by the sympathetic nerve endings [8-100]. In the liver, catecholamines are metabolized to the methylated products normetanephrine and metanephrine. Very little of the hormone reaches the brain, since the blood-brain barrier effectively excludes the brain with the exception of the hypothalamus [8-101].

Action of the Catecholamines

Catecholamines affect a variety of organs. The major response occurs in the heart and blood vessels with the production of an increased rate and force of cardiac contraction. Catecholamines affect arteriolar muscle as vasodilators in low doses and vasoconstrictors in higher doses. Respiration is enhanced, force of contraction of skeletal muscle is increased, and smooth muscle in general is stimulated. Hyperglycemia is produced by stimulation of hepatic glycogenolysis, and free fatty acids are released from adipose tissue into the serum. The duration of action of circulating catecholamine is extremely short, and most effects last for approximately one minute [8-102].

Regulation of Adrenal Medullary Secretion

The rapid tissue uptake of catecholamines from the plasma and the secretion of catecholamines by sympathetic nerve endings produce large variations in arterial and venous levels of hormones. Therefore, measurement of the level of catecholamine secretion by sampling circulating blood has been difficult. Early studies showed elevation of epinephrine and norepinephrine levels in patients with serious operation or severe trauma. Patients with acute infections also showed elevation of catecholamine levels [8-103]. The fact that catecholamine secretion is stimulated by pain, changes in temperature, and emotional states also makes analysis difficult. It is clear that secretion occurs due to stimulation of the carotid sinus by hypotension [8-104]. Thus adrenal medullary catecholamines represent an important limb of the closed-loop feedback system for arterial blood pressure regulation.

Alterations in blood-gas levels apparently directly affect secretory rates of catecholamines. Hypoxia results in an increase in secretion of both epinephrine and norepinephrine [8-105], and severe hypercarbia results in massive outpouring of hormone [8-106]. These studies also confirm the fact that circulating levels may not represent secretory rates [8-105]. It would appear that the most appropriate methodology for measurement of secretion is either adrenal vein cannulation or the measurement of metabolic products excreted in the urine [8-107].

Adrenal Medullary Insufficiency

Insufficiency of adrenal medullary secretion is almost never encountered in human patients with intact adrenals. Patients with bilateral adrenalectomy appear to be able to maintain the blood pressure by means other than medullary catecholamine secretion. Medullary replacement therapy is not required providing cortical replacement therapy is adequate.

Catecholamine Excess—Pheochromocytoma

Hypersecretion of adrenal medullary hormones occurs due to neoplasm of the chromaffin cells in the adrenal medulla or in other areas of the sympathetic nervous system. Most patients with pheochromocytoma exhibit hypertension, either sustained or paroxysmal, and from this the presence of the tumor may be suspected. However, in some patients pheochromocytoma may be occult, and massive secretion of catecholamines may occur only upon stimulation by drugs, anxiety, hemorrhage, or stress. If such patients come to operation undiagnosed, the mortality can be as high as 50 per cent [8-108]. The possibility that a pheochromocytoma may be present in any hypertensive patient must be kept in mind to prevent such untoward occurrence.

Analysis of excreted metabolic products of the catecholamines can be performed with accuracy and elevated levels indicate the presence of a pheochromocytoma [8-109]. When the presence of such a tumor is documented, appropriate therapy will make the operative procedure essentially safe. Therapy includes restoration of the abnormally decreased blood volume [8-110], and the proper preoperative use of alpha blockade [8-111], and beta blockade [8-112].

PITUITARY

The central controlling function of the hypothalamo-hypophyseal system has become clarified over the past 40 years, since the early studies of the neural and vascular connections between these two structures [8-113, 8-114, 8-115].

Posterior Lobe

The posterior lobe of the pituitary, or the neurohypophysis, releases hormones synthesized in the supraoptic and paraventricular nuclei of the hypothalamus. The most important of these hormones are oxytocin and vasopressin. The importance of vasopressin in the maintenance of normal plasma osmolarity and the regulation of water resorption by the kidney has been discussed. Oxytocin acts to produce milk ejection from the mammary gland and to increase smooth-muscle contracture, especially that of the uterus.

Anterior Lobe

The anterior pituitary, or adenohypophysis, produces a number of vital trophic hormones which include the three gonadotropins, follicle stimulating hormone (FHS), luteinizing hormone (LH), and prolactin. Also produced are adrenocorticotrophic hormone (ACTH) and thyroid stimulating hormone (TSH). In addition the adenohypophysis produces growth hormone. These hormones are released from specific cells in the adenohypophysis following stimulation by chemical mediators secreted in the hypothalamus and carried to the adenohypophyseal cells by the hypophyseal portal veins. Each one of these hormonal systems has its own closed loop feedback regulatory system.

Response to Trauma

Secretion of vasopressin by the posterior pituitary is stimulated by hypovolemia [8-116], hypotension, and excitation of pain receptors [8-117], all occurring frequently due to trauma.

The anterior pituitary releases increased amounts of ACTH during stress [8-91], presumably due to increase in hypothalamic production of adrenocorticotrophin-releasing factor [8-92].

Growth hormone production is elevated also by shock and trauma [8-118]. This elevation may explain some of the hypermetabolism noted in the injured patient.

TSH may be stimulated also in stress states. Radioactive iodine uptake by the thyroid is increased [8-31].

Pituitary Insufficiency

Although the primacy of the hypothalamo-hypophyseal system in the regulation of body endocrine balance is clear, the effects of pituitary insufficiency on body metabolism are mainly those of deficiencies in function of the endocrine end-organs themselves. Insufficiency of the posterior pituitary thus produces diabetes insipidus, with inability of the kidney to retain water appropriately. Anterior pituitary deficiency of mild degree first influences the gonadotropins, and thyroid and adrenal function may be quite normal. With a greater loss of anterior pituitary function, hypothyroidism may be present and adrenal function may be moderately normal, insufficiency being unmasked only by the stress of trauma. Severe or panhypopituitarism results in hypothyroidism and adrenal cortical insufficiency.

Treatment of Pituitary Insufficiency

Patients with clear-cut panhypopituitarism must be supported by the administration of vasopressin to correct the water resorption abnormality of diabetes insipidus, and by the administration of appropriate doses of thyroid hormone and corticosteroids. In such patients appropriate increases in corticosteroid support will be needed during the period of stress of trauma or operation. The patient who shows only mild to moderate hypothyroidism of pituitary origin may not need support with corticosteroids under ordinary conditions, but may develop adrenal insufficiency following trauma or operation. It is therefore very important in such a patient to determine whether the hypothyroidism is primary or secondary, and thus to determine the state of function of the pituitary [8-119].

DETECTION OF SECONDARY HYPOTHYROIDISM

Differentiation between primary and secondary hypothyroidism may be made by measurement of the circulating TSH level. This level should be elevated in primary hypothyroidism and decreased in hypopituitarism. Measurement of I-131 uptake and protein-bound iodine levels before and after stimulation of the thyroid with injections of TSH will also help to differentiate the two types. In pituitary hypothyroidism, I-131 uptake and protein bound iodine levels will be increased following TSH administration.

TESTS FOR ADRENAL CORTICAL FUNCTION

Determination of the state of the adrenal cortex is also of vital importance in such a patient and the response to intravenous administration of ACTH is the method which may be used to evaluate adrenal cortical adequacy. Twenty-five units of ACTH in saline are given intravenously in 8 hours on each of two successive days. Twenty-four-hour urine specimens are obtained prior to the infusions and on each day of the test infusion. A three- to fivefold increase in urinary 17-hydroxycorticoids is produced on the first day in the normal individual. In patients with secondary adrenal cortical insufficiency due to hypopituitarism there is a slight increase on the first day with a larger increase on the second day. In patients with primary adrenal cortical insufficiency no increase in 17-hydroxycorticoids is produced.

Appropriate therapy with thyroid hormone and corticosteroids must be administered to enable the patient with pituitary insufficiency to recover from the stress of sepsis, trauma, or operation. Diabetes insipidus requires specific therapy with vasopressin. Usually aldosterone release is not abnormal since ACTH is not involved in the release of aldosterone from the adrenal cortex under most conditions. Sodium metabolism, therefore, will usually be normal in these patients.

REFERENCES

8-1. Krahl, M. E.: The action of insulin on cells. New York, Academic Press, 1961.

8-2. Tepperman, J.: Metabolic and endocrine physiology. Chicago, Ill., Year Book Medical Publishers, 1962.

8-3. Yalow, R. S., and Berson, S. A.: Immunoassay of endogenous plasma insulin in man. J. Clin. Invest. 39:1157, 1960.

8-4. Yalow, R. S., and Berson, S. A.: Plasma insulin concentrations in nondiabetic and early diabetic subjects: determinations by a new sensitive immuno-assay technic. Diabetes 9:254, 1960.

8-5. Berson, S. A., and Yalow, R. S.: Some current controversies in diabetes research. Diabetes 14:549, 1965.

8-6. Conn, J. W.: Hypertension, the potassium ion and impaired carbohydrate tolerance. New Engl. J. Med. 273:1135, 1965.

8-7. Siperstein, M. D., Unger, R. H., and Madison, L. L.: Studies of muscle capillary basement membranes in normal subjects, diabetic, and prediabetic patients. J. Clin. Invest. 47:1973, 1968.

8-8. Kimmelstien, P., and Wilson, C.: Intercapillary lesions in the glomeruli of the kidney. Am. J. Path. 12:83, 1936.

8-9. Fahr, T.: Uber glomerulosklerose. Virchows Arch. f. Path. Anat. 309:16, 1942.

8-10. Forster, H. W., Jr.: Ocular diabetes. Med. Clin. N. Amer. 40:1641, 1956.

8-11. Pirort, J.: Diabetic neuropathy: A metabolic or a vascular disease? Diabetes. 14:1, 1965.

8-12. Ellenberg, M.: Long-term problems: diabetic neuropathy, in T. A. Danowski (ed.), Diabetes Mellitus: Diagnosis and Treatment. New York, American Diabetes Assoc., 1964, p. 171.

8-13. Brayton, R. G., Stokes, P. E., Schwertz, M. S., and Louria, D. B.: Effect of alcohol and various diseases on leukocyte mobilization, phagocytosis and intracellular bacterial killing. New Engl. J. Med. 282:123, 1970.

8-14. Drachman, R. H., Root, R. K., and Wood, W. B., Jr.: Studies on the effect of experimental non-ketotic diabetes mellitus on antibacterial defense. 1: Demonstration of a defect in phagocytosis. J. Exp. Med. 124:227, 1972.

8-15. Cruickshank, A. H.: Resistance to infection in the alloxan-diabetic rabbit. J. Path. Bact. 67:323, 1954.

8-16. Galloway, J. A., and Shuman, C. R.: Diabetes and surgery. Am. J. Med. 34:177, 1963.

8-17. Steinke, J.: Management of diabetes in the surgical patient. Med. Clin. N. Amer. 55:939, 1971.

8-18. Samols, E., Tyler, J., Marri, G., and Marks, V.: Stimulation of glucagon secretion by oral glucose. Lancet 2:1257, 1965.

8-19. Unger, R. H.: Glucagon physiology and pathophysiology. New Engl. J. Med. 285:443, 1971.

8-20. Wool, I. G., and Krahl, M. E.: Incorporation of C^{14}-histidine into protein of isolated diaphrams: Interaction of fasting glucose and insulin. Am. J. Physiol. 197:367, 1959.

8-21. Unger, R. H., Ohneda, A., Aguilar-Parada, E., and Eisentraut, A. M.: The role of aminogenic glucagon secretion in blood glucose homeostasis. J. Clin. Invest. 48:810, 1969.

8-22. Unger, R. H., Aguilar-Parada, E., Miller, W. A., and Eisentraut, A. M.: Studies of pancreatic alpha-cell function in normal and diabetic subjects. J. Clin. Invest. 48:837, 1970.

8-23. Muller, W. A., Faloona, G. R., Aguilar-Parada, E., and Unger, R. H.: Abnormal alpha-cell function in diabetes. New Engl. J. Med. 283:109, 1970.

8-24. Kyle, L. H., Ball, M. F., and Doolan, P. D.: Effect of thyroid hormone on body composition in myxedema and obesity. New Engl. J. Med. 275:12, 1966.

8-25. Gold, H. K., Spann, J. F., Jr., and Braunwald, E.: Effect of alterations in the thyroid state on the intrinsic contractile properties of isolated rat skeletal muscle. J. Clin. Invest. 49:849, 1970.

8-26. Kontos, H. A., Shapiro, W., Mauck, H. P., Jr., Richardson, D. W., Patterson, J. L., Jr., and Sharpe, A. R., Jr.: Mechanism of certain abnormalities of the circulation to the limbs in thyrotoxicosis. J. Clin. Invest. 44:947, 1965.

8-27. Massey, D. G., Becklake, M. R., McKenzie, J. M., and Bates, D. V.: Circulatory and ventilatory response to exercise in thyrotoxicosis. New Engl. J. Med. 276:1104, 1967.

8-28. Brewster, W. R., Jr., Isaacs, J. R., Osgood, P. F., and King, T. L.: The hemodynamic and metabolic interrelationships in the activity of epinephrine, norepinephrine and the thyroid hormones. Circulation 13:1, 1956.

8-29. Ingbar, S. H.: Management of Emergencies: IX. Thyrotoxic storm. New Engl. J. Med. 274:1252, 1966.

8-30. DeNiord, R. N., Jr., and Hayes, M. A.: Endocrine interrelations concerned with the postoperative renal response to a water load. Surg. Gynec. Obst. 98:617, 1954.

8-31. Goldenberg, I. S., Lutwak, L., Rosenbaum, P. J., and Hayes, M. A.: Thyroid-adrenocortical interrelations following operation. Surg. Gynec. Obst. 98:516, 1954.

8-32. Wilson, O., Hedner, P., Laurell, S., Nosslin, B., Rerup, C., and Rosengren, E.: Thyroid and adrenal response to acute cold exposure in man. J. App. Physiol., 28:543, 1970.

8-33. Nicoloff, J. T., Fisher, D. A., and Appleman, M. D., Jr.: The role of glucocorticoids in the regulation of thyroid function in man. J. Clin. Invest. 49:1922, 1970.

8-34. Catt, K. J.: The thyroid gland. Lancet 1:1383, 1970.

8-35. Copp, D. H., and Davison, G. F.: Direct humoral control of para- thyroid function in the dog. Proceedings of the Society for Ex- perimental Biology and Medicine. 107:342, 1961.

8-36. Sherwood, L. M., and Potts, J. T.: Evaluation by radioimmunoassay of factors controlling the secretion of parathyroid hormone. Na- ture 209:52, 1966.

8-37. Kaplan, E. L., Hill, B. J., Loke, S., and Peskin, G. W.: Acid-base balance and parathyroid function: Metabolic alkalosis and hyper- parathyroidism. Surgery 70:198, 1971.

8-38. Sherwood, L. M.: Relative importance of parathyroid hormone and thyrocalcitonin in calcium homeostasis. New Engl. J. Med. 278:663, 1968.

8-39. Munson, P. L.: Studies on the role of the parathyroids in calcium and phosphorous metabolism. Ann. N.Y. Acad. Sci. 60:776, 1955.

8-40. Wells, H.: Proc. 3rd Parathyroid Conference, Mt. Gabriel, Quebec, Canada. Oct. 16–20, 1967. Excerpta Med., 1967.

8-41. Chase, L. R., and Aurbach, G. D.: Parathyroid function and the renal excretion of 3',5'-adenylic acid. Nat. Acad. Sci. 58:518, 1967.

8-42. Cope, O.: The Story of hyperparathyroidism at the Massachusetts General Hospital. New Engl. J. Med. 274:1174, 1966.

8-43. Egdahl, R. H.: Surgery of the parathyroid glands. Surg. Gynec. Obst. 130:901, 1970.

8-44. Goldsmith, R. S.: Hyperparathyroidism. New Engl. J. Med. 281: 367, 1969.

8-45. Berson, S. A., and Yalow, R. S.: Parathyroid hormone in plasma in adenomatous hyperparathyroidism, uremia, and bronchogenic carcinoma. Science 154:907, 1966.

8-46. Haff, R. C., Black, W. C., and Ballinger, W. F., II.: Primary hyper- parathyroidism: changing clinical, surgical and pathologic aspects. Ann. Surg. 171:85, 1970.

8-47. Rogers, H. M., Keating, F. R., Jr., Molock, C. G., and Barker, N. W.: Primary hypertrophy and hyperplasia of the parathyroid glands associated with duodenal ulcer. Arch. Intern. Med. 79:307, 1947.

8-48. Ellis, C., and Nicoloff, D. M.: Hyperparathyroidism and peptic ulcer disease. Arch. Surg. 96:114, 1968.

8-49. Paloyan, E., Lawrence, A. M., Straus, F. H., II., Paloyan, D., Har- per, P. V., and Cummings, D.: Alpha-cell hyperplasia in calcific pancreatitis associated with hyperparathyroidism. JAMA 200:97, 1967.

8-50. Lemann, J., Jr., and Donatelli, A.: Calcium intoxication due to primary hyperparathyroidism. Ann. Intern. Med. 60:447, 1964.

8-51. Goldsmith, R. S., and Ingbar, S. H.: Inorganic phosphate treatment of hypercalcemia of diverse etiologies. New Engl. J. Med. 274:1, 1966.

8-52. Chakmakjian, Z. H., and Bethune, J. E.: Sodium sulfate treatment of hypercalcemia. New Engl. J. Med. 275:862, 1966.

8-53. Levy, R. I.: Effect of forced saline diuresis with ethacrycic acid in hypercalcemia. Am. Soc. Nephrol. 1969.

8-54. Munson, P. L., Tashjian, A. H., Jr., and Levine, L.: Evidence for parathyroid hormone in nonparathyroid tumors associated with hypercalcemia. Cancer Res. 25:1062, 1965.

8-55. Sherwood, L. M., O'Riordan, J. L. H., Aurbach, G. D., and Potts, J. T., Jr.: Production of parathyroid hormone by nonparathyroid tumors. J. Clin. Endocr. Metab. 27:140, 1967.

8-56. Goldsmith, R. S.: Differential diagnosis of hypercalcemia. New Engl. J. Med. 274:674, 1966.

8-57. Kleinfeld, G.: A complication in estrogen therapy of metastatic breast cancer. JAMA 181:1137, 1962.

8-58. McLean, F. C.: The parathyroid hormone and bone. Clin. Ortho. 9:46, 1957.

8-59. Ireland, A. W., Clubb, J. S., Neale, F. C., Posen, S., and Reeve, T. S.: The calciferol requirements of patients with surgical hypoparathyroidism. Ann. Intern. Med. 69:81, 1968.

8-60. Tashjian, A. H., Jr., Barowsky, N. J., and Jensen, D. K.: Thyrotropin-releasing hormone: direct evidence for stimulation of prolactin production by pituitary cells in culture. Biochem. Biophys. Res. Commun. 43:516, 1971.

8-61. Pearse, A. G. E., and Carvalheira, A. F.: Cytochemical evidence for an ultimobranchial origin of rodent thyroid C cells. Nature 214:929, 1967.

8-62. Foster, G. V., Baghdiantz, A., Kumar, M. A., Slack, E., Soliman, H. A., and MacIntyre, I.: Thyroid origin of calcitonin. Nature 202:1303, 1964.

8-63. Buckwalter, J. A., Soper, R. T., Davies, J., and Mason, E. E.: Postoperative hypoparathyroidism. Surg. Gynec. Obst. 101:657, 1955.

8-64. Melby, J. C.: Assessment of adrenocortical function. New Engl. J. Med. 285:735, 1971.

8-65. Salassa, R. M., Bennett, W. A., Keating, F. R., Jr., and Sprague, R. G.: Postoperative adrenal cortical insufficiency. JAMA 152:1509, 1953.

8-66. Hayes, M. A.: Surgical treatment as complicated by prior adrenocortical steroid therapy. Surgery 40:945, 1956.

8-67. Howland, W. S., Schweizer, O., Boyan, C. P., and Dotto, A. C.:

Treatment of adrenal cortical insufficiency during surgical procedures. JAMA 160:1271, 1956.

8-68. Webb, W. R., Degreli, I. U., Hardy, J. D., and Unal, M.: Cardiovascular responses in adrenal insufficiency. Surgery 58:273, 1965.

8-69. Verrier, R. L., Rovetto, M. J., and Lefer, A. M.: Blood volume and myocardial function in adrenal insufficiency. Am. J. Physiol. 217:1559, 1969.

8-70. Gann, D. S., and Egdahl, R. H.: Responses of adrenal corticosteroid secretion to hypotension and hypovolemia. J. Clin. Invest. 44:1, 1965.

8-71. Marks, L. J., King, D. W., and McCarthy, H. F.: Physiological role of cortisol in the plasma volume response to hemorrhage. Surgery 61:422, 1967.

8-72. McNeil, I. F., Dixon, J. P., and Moore, F. D.: The effect of hemorrhage and hormones on the partition of body water: III. The effects of hemorrhage and corticosteroids on fluid partition in the adrenalectomized dog. J. Surg. Res. 111:344, 1963.

8-73. Beisel, W., and Rapoport, M. I.: Interrelations between adrenocortical functions and infectious illness. New Engl. J. Med. 280:541, 1969.

8-74. Munck, A.: Glucocorticoid inhibition of glucose uptake by peripheral tissues: old and new evidence, molecular mechanisms, and physiological significance. Perspectives in Biology and Medicine, Winter 1971, p. 265.

8-75. O'Malley, B. W.: Mechanisms of action of steroid hormones. New Engl. J. Med. 284:368, 1971.

8-76. Bongiovanni, A. M., and Root, A. W.: The adrenogenital syndrome. New Engl. J. Med. 268:1283, 1963.

8-77. Cushing, H.: The pituitary body and its disorders. Philadelphia, Lippincott, 1912.

8-78. Albright, F.: Cushing's Syndrome. The Harvey lectures series. 38:132, 1942–43.

8-79. Glenn, F., and Mannix, H., Jr.: Diagnosis and prognosis of Cushing's Syndrome. Surg. Gynec. Obst. 126:765, 1968.

8-80. Egdahl, R. H.: Surgery of the adrenal gland. New Engl. J. Med. 278:939, 1968.

8-81. Kaplan, N. M., and Cook, R.: The biosynthesis of adrenal steroids: Effects of angiotensin II, adrencorticotropin, and potassium. J. Clin. Invest. 44:2029, 1965.

8-82. Blair-West, J. R., Coghland, J. P., Denton, D. A., Munro, J. A., Peterson, R. E., and Wintour, M.: Humoral stimulation of adrenal cortical secretion. J. Clin. Invest. 41:1606, 1962.

8-83. Rhamy, R. K., McCoy, R. M., Scott, H. W., Jr., Fishman, L. M., Michelakis, A. M., and Liddle, G. W.: Primary aldosteronism: experience with current diagnostic criteria and surgical treatment in fourteen patients. Ann. Surg. 167:718, 1968.

8-84. Conn, J. W.: Plasma renin activity in primary aldosteronism: Importance in differential diagnosis and in research of essential hypertension. JAMA 190:220, 1964.

8-85. Cannon, W. B.: Bodily changes in pain, hunger, fear and rage. New York, Appleton, 1915.

8-86. Albright, F.: Cushing's syndrome, its pathological physiology. Harvey Lect. 38:133, 1942–43.

8-87. Selye, H.: The general adaptation syndrome and the disease of adaptation. J. Clin. Endocrin. 6:117, 1946.

8-88. Moore, F. D., Steenburg, R. W., Ball, M. R., Wilson, G. M., and Myrden, J. A.: Studies in surgical endocrinology: the urinary excretion of 17-hydroxycorticoids, and associated metabolic changes, in cases of soft tissue trauma of varying severity and in bone trauma. Ann. Surg. 141:145, 1965.

8-89. Steenburg, R. W., Lennihan, R., and Moore, F. D.: Studies in surgical endocrinology. II. The free blood 17-hydroxycorticoids in surgical patients: their relation to urine steroids, metabolism and convalescence. Ann. Surg. 143:180, 1956.

8-90. Hume, D. M., Bell, C. C., and Bartter, F.: Direct measurement of adrenal secretion during operative trauma and convalescence. Surgery 52:174, 1962.

8-91. Cooper, C. E., and Nelson, D. H.: ACTH levels in plasma in preoperative and surgically stressed patients. J. Clin. Invest. 41:1566, 1962.

8-92. Anderson, E.: Adrenocorticotrophin-releasing hormone in peripheral blood: increase during stress. Science 152:379, 1966.

8-93. Galante, M., Rukes, M., Forsham, P. H., and Bell, H. G.: The use of corticotropin, cortisone and hydrocortisone in general surgery. Surg. Clin. N. A., 34:1201, 1954.

8-94. Nelson, D. H.: Determining plasma and urinary corticosteroids: Normal values and clinical pitfalls. Postgrad. Med. 46:135, 1969.

8-95. Smilo, R. P., and Forsham, P. H.: Diagnostic approach to hypofunction and hyperfunction of the adrenal cortex. Post Grad. Med. 46:146, 1969.

8-96. Greenwood, F. C., Landon, J., and Stamp, T. C. B.: The plasma sugar, free fatty acid, cortisol, and growth hormone response to insulin. 1. In control subjects. J. Clin. Invest. 45:429, 1966.

8-97. Brostoff, J., James, V. H. T., and Landon, J.: Plasma corticosteroid and growth hormone response to lysine-vasopressin in man. J. Clin. Invest. Metab. 28:511, 1968.

8-98. Perlmutter, M.: Rapid test for adrenocortical insufficiency. JAMA 160:117, 1956.

8-99. Axelrod, J., Weil-Malherbe, H., and Tomchick, R.: the Physiological disposition of H³-epinephrine and its metabolite metanephrine. J. Pharmacol. Exper. Therap. 127:251, 1959.

8-100. Potter, L. T., and Axelrod, J.: Subcellular localization of cate-
        cholamines in tissues of the rat. J. Pharmacol. Exper. Therap.
        142:291, 1963.
8-101. Weil-Malherbe, H., Axelrod, J., and Tomchick, R.: Blood-brain
        barrier for adrenaline. Science 129:1226, 1959.
8-102. Wortma, R. J., Kopin, I. J., and Axelrod, J.: Thyroid function
        and the cardiac disposition of catecholamines. Endocrinology
        73:63, 1963.
8-103. Hammond, W. C., Aronow, L., and Moore, F. D.: Studies in surgi-
        cal endocrinology III: Plasma concentrations of epinephrine and
        norepinephrine in anesthesia, trauma and surgery, as measured
        by a modification of the method of Weil-Malherbe and Bone.
        Ann. Surg. 144:715, 1956.
8-104. Heymans, C.: Sur la régulation reflex du tonus vasomoteur et
        de l'adrénalinesécretion en rapport avec la pression arterielle.
        Compt. Ren. Soc. de Biol. 100:765, 1929.
8-105. Harrison, T. S., and Seaton, J.: Respiratory influences on the secre-
        tion of catecholamines. J. Surg. Res. 5:556, 1965.
8-106. Harrison, T. S., and Seaton, J.: The relative effects of hypoxia
        and hypercarbia on adrenal medullary secretion in anesthetized
        dogs. J. Surg. Rev. 5:560, 1965.
8-107. Wolf, R. L., Mendlowitz, M., Roboz, J., and Gitlow, S. E.: New
        rapid test for pheochromocytoma: urinary assay of normetaneph-
        rine, and 3-methoxy-4-hydroxyphenylglycol. JAMA 188:135,
        1964.
8-108. Apgar, V., and Papper, E. M.: Pheochromocytoma: anesthetic
        management during surgical treatment. Arch. Surg. 62:634, 1951.
8-109. Wolf, R. L., Mendlowitz, M. D., Roboz, J., and Gitlow, S. E.:
        Simultaneous urinary assays for the combined metanephrines
        and 3-methoxy-4-hydroxyphenylglycol in patients with pheochro-
        mocytoma and primary hypertension. New Engl. J. Med.
        273:1459, 1965.
8-110. Brunjes, S., Johns, V. J., Jr., and Crane, M. G.: Pheochromo-
        cytama: postoperative shock and blood volume. New Engl. J.
        Med. 262:393, 1960.
8-111. Glenn, F., and Mannix, H., Jr.: The surgical management of chro-
        maffin tumors. Ann. Surg. 167:619, 1968.
8-112. Prichard, B. N. C., and Ross, E. J.: Use of propranolol in conjunc-
        tion with alpha receptor blocking drugs in pheochromocytoma.
        Am. J. Cardiol. 18:394, 1966.
8-113. Wislock, G. B., and King, L. S.: The permeability of the hypophysis
        and hypothalamus to vital dyes, with a study of the hypophyseal
        vascular supply. Am. J. Anat. 58:421, 1936.
8-114. Rioch, D. M.: Neurophysiology of corpus striatum and globus palli-
        dus. Psychiatry 3:119, 1940.

8-115. Harris, G. W.: Neural control of the pituitary gland. London, Arnold, 1955.

8-116. Shane, L., and Travis, R. H.: Interrelations between the adrenal cortex and the posterior pituitary. Fed. Proc. 30:1378, 1971.

8-117. Moran, W. H., Jr., Miltenberger, F. W., and Shuayb, W. A., and Zimmerman, B.: The relationship of antidiuretic hormone secretion to surgical stress. Surgery 56:99, 1964.

8-118. Carey, L. C., Cloutier, C. T., and Lowery, B. D.: Growth hormone and adrenal cortical response to shock and trauma in the human. Ann. Surg. 174:451, 1971.

8-119. Dingman, J. F.: Pituitary function. New Engl. J. Med. 285:617, 1971.

9

AUTONOMIC NERVOUS SYSTEM

The autonomic nervous system is a regulatory mechanism which is involved in adjusting the function of almost all tissues of the body. The two main divisions are the sympathetic (adrenergic) and parasympathetic (cholinergic).

SYMPATHETIC NERVOUS SYSTEM

The sympathetic nervous system is best described as a part of the neuroendocrine mechanism, specifically the sympathoadrenal apparatus. This terminology indicates the extensive interrelationship between the sympathetic nervous system, the adrenal medulla, and the catecholamines.

General Function

Cannon described the sympathetic nervous system as a system which prepares the body for increased activity under emergency conditions [9-1]. It functions in an organized and total way. Sympathetic activity produces a coordinated change in body mechanisms. This change may be described as tending to reduce all activity which does not contribute to muscular function. Therefore actions of the sympathetic nervous system are to cause vasoconstriction in the viscera, and to inhibit motility of the gastrointestinal tract and secretion of most glands. In addition, sympathetic activity facilitates muscular effort. This is accomplished by an increase in the heart rate and the force of myocardial contraction, vasodilatation in skeletal muscle, activation of sweat glands, dilatation of bronchioles, and contraction of the spleen. An increase in adrenal secretion is caused which in turn mobilizes free fatty acid and increases glycogenolysis. To aid in this function and to emphasize the overall coordinated activity of sympathetic nervous system, the chemotransmitter norepinephrine which is released by sympthetic nerve endings spills over into the blood stream and reinforces sympathetic activity by being transported to alpha and beta adrenergic receptor sites.

Norepinephrine Metabolism

Norepinephrine is synthesized from tyrosine through a series of enzymatic reactions [9-2]. The major source of circulating norepinephrine in man is the sympathetic nerve ending and bilateral adrenalectomy fails to depress urinary excretion of norepinephrine [9-3]. By contrast, all of the epinephrine in the blood comes from the adrenal medulla and adrenalectomy causes a marked and rapid fall of greater than 80 per cent in urinary epinephrine [9-4].

Almost all of the norepinephrine and epinephrine present in tissue is located within highly specialized subcellular particles, or granules, within adrenergic nerves [9-5], and chromaffin cells [9-6]. Within these cells dopamine is oxidized to norepinephrine through the action of dopamine beta oxidase and storage of norepinephrine takes place. The presence of the hormone within the granule protects it from enzymatic destruction by monoamine oxidase [9-7].

Norepinephrine Secretion

Norepinephrine is released from sympathetic nerve endings continuously since arterial norepinephrine content is always less than that in the peripheral venous blood [9-8]. When the sympathetic nerves to an organ are stimulated, norepinephrine in increased amounts is released into the circulation. Pharmacologic or surgical blockade of sympathetic nerve transmission reduces the spontaneous release of norepinephrine from the organ so blockaded, but does not completely abolish it, indicating that there is some spontaneous sympathetic activity independent of nerve innervation [9-9].

Tissue Uptake of Catecholamine

Organ uptake of circulating catecholamines is proportional to the number of sympathetic nerve endings present in the tissue. Sympathetic nerves take up epinephrine from the circulation almost as efficiently as norepinephrine. Since epinephrine is synthesized only in the adrenal medulla, heart, and midbrain, most organs receive epinephrine from the circulation. Sympathetic denervation blocks uptake of epinephrine and norepinephrine from the blood.

Effects of Sympathetic Stimulation

The effects of sympathetic nerve stimulation are similar to those obtained by the injection of catecholamine. These effects are predominantly on the heart and cardiovascular system, inducing an increase in strength of contracture and heart rate. Some types of smooth muscle are caused to contract, such as skin arterioles and visceral vessels, whereas others are dilated, such as arterioles in skeletal muscle and bronchi. Two types of receptor sites have been postulated to account for these two effects of catecholamines: alpha receptors for smooth-muscle contraction and beta receptors for smooth muscle relaxation [9-10]. In addition, catecholamine release increases glycogenolysis, causes the release of fatty acids, and produces relaxation in intestinal smooth muscle [9-11].

Operative Sympathectomy

Interruption of the function of the adrenergic nervous system in man by surgery has been carried out to treat a variety of conditions, usually those presumed to be associated with vasospasm. Examples are hypertension and arterial insufficiency. The predominant effects of such adrenergic ablation appear to be a decrease of arteriolar resistance and an increase in vascular capacitance. Sweating is also abolished. Grimson et al reported the effects of a variety of operative sympathectomies ranging in extent up to bilateral removal from T-1 through L-3 [9-12, 9-13]. In these patients postural hypotension was severe, presumably due to the removal of vasoconstrictor effect in the lower extremitites. A somewhat less extensive resection, however, with bilateral removal from the stellate ganglion through L-1 resulted in little postural hypotension. Expansion of the vascular volume with blood transfusion was required to stabilize the patient following removal of the second sympathetic chain [9-12]. Other effects noted in these patients were unexplained hyperpyrexia (removal of sweating capacity?) and nasal congestion due to loss of vasoconstriction of the nasal mucous membrane.

Pharmacologic Sympathectomy

Alteration of adrenergic activity by the administration of drugs has become more common in recent years. These drugs fall into several categories. Some agents interfere with the uptake of norepinephrine into sympathetic nerve endings. Such drugs are cocaine and chlorpromazine [9-9]. Certain agents cause the release of norepinephrine from the sympathetic nerve endings. If such norepinephrine release is in the active form, an enhancement of sympathetic activity occurs. Examples of such agents are tyramine, ephedrin, and amphetamine. Reserpine depletes the brain and sympathetically innervated organs of most of their catecholamines by a direct effect on the storage vesicle. Enhancement of sympathetic activity does not accompany this release because the norepinephrine is deaminated before leaving the nerve ending [9-14]. Following depletion of norepinephrine storage by reserpine, sympathetic nerve endings remain unable to respond in a normal fashion until such stores are repleted. Other agents block the release of tissue norepinephrine. Examples of these are bretylium and guanethidine. The ganglionic blocking agents interfere with the release of norepinephrine by blocking the transmission of preganglionic nerve impulses through the ganglion to the nerve ending. Monoamine oxidase inhibitors act to prevent the interneuronal metabolism of norepinephrine [9-7].

Function in Stress

The function and responsiveness of the sympathoadrenal system appears to be maintained even in the presence of severe chronic depletion and serious acute stress. Output of noradrenaline is increased manyfold in stressful states and conditions of hypovolemia. It may be that in severe continuing stress, such as that caused by severe burns, the sympathoadrenal system becomes unable to respond adequately. Goodall and coworkers have shown subnormal urinary output of epinephrine and subnormal epinephrine content of the adrenal in such patients [9-15]. These investigators have shown that norepinephrine excretion also is subnormal in certain patients under burn stress. Sympathetic nerves in these patients contained a subnormal amount of stored norepinephrine [9-16]. Such depletion of catecholamines occurred more frequently in patients who went on to die of their burn injury. It would appear possible, therefore, that failure of the sympathoadrenal system may occur under unusual conditions of prolonged stress.

PARASYMPATHETIC NERVOUS SYSTEM

Parasympathetic activity, mediated by the craniosacral outflow of cranial nerves 3, 7, 9, 10, and sacral segments 2, 3, and 4, produces a variety of effects which are of local importance, but which form no integrated generalized pattern.

General Function

Activity of the cranial parasympathetics is directed toward conservation of body resources. Such action includes constriction of the pupil, slowing of the heart, and constriction of the bronchi. Function of the alimentary tract is enhanced by stimulation of salivation, increase in peristalsis, and relaxation of intestinal sphincters. In addition, secretion of the intestinal mucous glands and the associated glands such as the pancreas, is stimulated.

The sacral outflow aids in elimination of waste products from the body and causes contraction of the bladder detrusor muscle with relaxation of the urethral sphincter. Increase in colon motility is produced and vasodilatation occurs in the genitalia.

Acetylcholine

In keeping with the local effects of parasympathetic activity, the chemotransmitter acetylcholine is immediately destroyed upon produc-

tion by the enzyme cholinesterase, and there is no spill over of acetylcholine into the general circulation.

Parasympathectomy

Loss of function of the parasympathetic cranial outflow in man
has essentially been confined to surgical division of the vagus nerves
below the level of the hilus of the lung. This produces denervation of
all of the lower esophagus, small intestine, and large intestine to the
mid-transverse colon. It also interrupts vagal stimulation of the acces-
sory digestive organs, the liver, biliary tract, and pancreas. The effect
of gastric vagotomy has been thoroughly studied. This procedure causes
a decrease in acid production due to interruption of vagal stimulation
of parietal cells, a decrease in gastric motility, and failure of relaxation
of the pylorus. Extragastric effects include delayed emptying of the gall-
bladder with some dilatation, and a possible increase in the incidence
of gallstones [9-17, 9-18].

Studies of pancreatic function after vagotomy have shown a variable effect with a decrease in secretory response to food and secretin
[9-19] reported by some investigators. In other studies pancreatic secretion appears to be normal [9-20].

The motility of the intestinal tract appears to be primarily affected,
with some patients showing atonicity of the esophagus [9-21]. The small
intestine shows decreased contractility with some dilatation [9-22, 9-23],
and intestinal villi appear to be decreased [9-24]. Diarrhea has been
the most disabling symptom in patients with total subhilar vagotomy,
occurring in approximately 10 per cent of patients [9-25, 9-26].

Complete autonomic denervation of the gastrointestinal tract by
thoracolumbar sympathectomy and vagotomy appears to interfere little
with normal function in man [9-27]. The vagotomy effect of gastric hypomotility appears to predominate and some patients show diarrhea.
Normal sensations of appetite, hunger, nausea, and heartburn are apparently preserved.

Interruption of the sacral outflow of the parasympathetic system
interferes with normal detrusor function in the bladder, and with rectal
and lower colonic contracture. Sphincter relaxation is interferred with.
Interval emptying by abdominal pressure and enemata can occur, however, as in a "cord bladder" [9-28]. Ejaculation is abolished in the male.

Spontaneous decrease in parasympathetic function does not appear
to be a clinically encountered condition. Certain unexplained "func-

tional" obstructive conditions of the large and small intestine are encountered, however, where mechanical lesions are absent. In these conditions abnormality or imbalance of sympathetic and parasympathetic innervation may play a part [9-29, 9-30, 9-31, 9-32].

REFERENCES

9-1. Cannon, W. B.: The wisdom of the body. 2nd ed. New York, Norton, 1939.

9-2. Nagatsu, T., Levitt, M., and Udenfriend, S.: Tyrosine hydroxylase—the initial step in nonepinephrine biosynthesis. J. Biol. Chem. 239:2910, 1964.

9-3. Von Euler, U. S., Franksson, C., and Hellstrom, J.: Adrenaline and noradrenaline output in urine after unilateral and bilateral adrenalectomy in man. Acta Physiol. Scand. 31:1, 1954.

9-4. Lund, A.: Release of adrenaline and noradrenaline from the suprarenal gland. Acta Pharmacol. et Toxicol. 7:309, 1951.

9-5. Von Euler, U. S., and Hillarp, N.-A.: Evidence for the presence of noradrenaline in submicroscopic structures of adrenergic axons. Nature 177:44, 1956.

9-6. Blaschko, H., and Welch, A. D.: Localization of adrenaline in cytoplasmic particles of the bovine adrenal medulla. Arch. f. Exper. Path. u Pharmakol. 219:17, 1953.

9-7. Kopin, I. J.: Storage and metabolism of catecholamines: The role of monoamine oxidase. Pharmacol. Rev. 16:179, 1964.

9-8. Von Euler, U. S., and Heller, H. (eds.): Comparative endocrinology. New York, Academic Press, 1963, pp. 258–290.

9-9. Hertting, G., Potter, L. T., and Axelrod, J.: Effect of decentralization and ganglionic blocking agents on the spontaneous release of H³-norepinephrine. J. Pharmacol. Exper. Therap. 136:289, 1962.

9-10. Ahlquist, R. P.: Adrenergic drugs. In V. A. Drill, (ed.), Pharmacology in medicine, a collaborative textbook. 2nd ed. New York, McGraw-Hill, 1958, pp. 378–407.

9-11. Wurtman, R. J.: Catecholamines. New Engl. J. Med. 273:637, 1965.

9-12. Grimson, K. S., Orgain, E. S., Anderson, B., and D'Angelo, G. J.: Total thoracic and partial to total lumbar sympathectomy, splanchnicectomy and celiac ganglionectomy for hypertension. Ann. Surg. 138:532, 1953.

9-13. Evans, J. A., Poppen, J. L., and Tobias, J. B.: Relief of angina pectoris by sympathectomy. JAMA 144:1432, 1950.

9-14. Kopin, I. J., and Gordon, E. K.: Metabolism of norepinephrine-H³ released by tyramine and reserpine. J. Pharmacol. Exper. Therap. 138:351, 1962.

9-15. Goodall, McC., and Haynes, B. W., Jr.: Adrenal medullary insufficiency in severe thermal burn. J. Clin. Invest. 39:1927, 1960.

9-16. Goodall, McC., and Moncrief, J. A.: Sympathetic nerve depletion in severe thermal injury. Ann. Surg. 162:983, 1965.

9-17. Cox, H. T., Doherty, J. F., and Kerr, D. F.: Changes in the gall bladder after elective gastric surgery. Lancet. 1:764, 1958.

9-18. Johnson, F. E., and Boyden, E. A.: The effect of double vagotomy on the motor activity of the human gall bladder. Surgery 32:591, 1952.

9-19. Pfeffer, R. B., Stephenson, H. E., and Hinton, J. W.: The effect of thoracolumbar sympathectomy and vagus resection on pancreatic function in man. Ann. Surg. 136:585, 1952.

9-20. White, T. T., Lenninger, S. G., Elmslie, R. G., and Magee, D. F.: Effect of truncal and selective vagotomy on duodenal aspirates in man. Ann. Surg. 164:257, 1966.

9-21. Postlethwait, R. W., Kim, S. K., and Dillon, M. L.: Esophageal complications of vagotomy. Surg. Gynec. Obst. 128:481, 1969.

9-22. Christeinsen, J.: The controls of gastrointestinal movements: Some old and new views. New Engl. J. Med. 285:85, 1971.

9-23. Issac, F., Ottoman, R. E., and Weinberg, J. A.: Roentgen studies of the upper gastrointestinal tract in vagotomy. Am. J. Roentgenol. 63:66, 1950.

9-24. Ballinger, W. F., II.: The small intestine following vagotomy. Surg. Gynec. Obst. 116:115, 1963.

9-25. Griffith, C. A.: Selective gastric vagotomy. West J. Surg. Gynec. Obst. 70:175, 1962.

9-26. Herrington, J. L., Jr., Edwards, W. H., Carter, J. H., and Sawyer, J. L.: Treatment of severe postvagotomy diarrhea by reversed jejunal segment. Ann. Surg. 168:522, 1968.

9-27. Bingham, J. R., and Ingelfinger, F. J.: Effect of combined sympathectomy and vagectomy of the gastrointestinal tract. JAMA 146:1406, 1951.

9-28. Localio, S. A., Francis, K. C., and Rossano, P. G.: Abdominosacral resection of sacrococcygeal chordoma. Ann. Surg. 166:394, 1967.

9-29. Zimmerman, L. M.: Spastic ileus. Surg. Gynec. Obst. 50:721, 1930.

9-30. Ogilvie, H.: Large-intestine colic due to sympathetic deprivation. B.M.J. 2:671, 1948.

9-31. Netto, A. C., Haddad, J., De Azevedo, P. A. V., and Raia, A.: Etiology, pathogenesis, and treatment of acquired megacolon. Surg. Gynec. Obst. 114:602, 1962.

9-32. Wanebo, H., Mathewson, C., and Conolly, B.: Pseudo-obstruction of the colon. Surg. Gynec. Obst. 133:44, 1971.

10
EMOTIONAL FACTORS

"The effects to the psyche . . . can function as etiologic agents, obscure the diagnosis, influence the pre- and postoperative course, precipitate complications, interfere with convalescence, and even prevent the complete recovery of the surgical patient."   [10-1]

EMOTIONAL IMPACT OF OPERATION

A surgical operation is usually perceived by the patient as a threat to normal existence. The seriousness of the threat depends upon the magnitude of the projected procedure, as perceived by the patient, and upon any specific unwanted results of the procedure, such as amputation or disfigurement. The timing of the occurrence is important. An acute injury produces an intense stress reaction as there is no time for psychic preparation, whereas an operation needed in the course of a chronic disease, as in ulcerative colitis or congestive heart failure, may be seen as a positive experience.

The threat in some ways resembles other types of life catastrophe or disaster. However, it is directed specifically toward the person, and carrys with it the possibility of suffering and pain, bodily damage or mutilation, and death. The emotional reaction to such stress, therefore, becomes an integral part of the patient's response to trauma and operation.

In some individuals the emotional reaction may be extremely complicated. The illness may be part of the life adjustment of the patient, and removal or correction of the disease process may precipitate a crisis of adjustment [10-2]. These individuals often become seriously depressed after recovery from operation. In many such patients, significant symptoms may continue in the postoperative period.

PHASES OF STRESS OF OPERATION

Reactions to surgical operations, like reactions to other threatening life situations vary as the threat is seen as a distant problem, an immediate problem, or a past experience. In most individuals anxiety grows as the operation approaches. Fear and worry are maximal at the time of operation and postoperative reactions of victimization may occur [10-3]. Many varieties of reaction occur within these phases, depending on the seriousness of the operation, on the individual personality, and on the cultural background. The most important factor in the determination of the patient's response to the stress of any operation is the previous personality state and the relationship of the current stressful situation to patterns of previous traumatic conditioning.

PATTERNS OF RESPONSE

Regression

A tendency toward regression to more childlike behavior is frequently seen. This tendency takes different forms in different individuals, depending on emotional responses originally elicited and reinforced during stress episodes of childhood. The patient may become overly sensitized to his own feelings. Natural reactions of fear and distaste may be interpreted as aggressive by the patient, and guilt feelings about such aggression may be generated. In addition, the patient may interpret the behavior of others as aggressive in nature.

The overriding tendency, as in childhood, is to curry the favor of the surgeon, as an authority figure, and thereby decrease any punishment for aggressive reactions. The surgeon must be aware of these feelings in the patient. A wish to please the authority figure can help the patient make decisions which achieve a good result. However, abuse of this emotional state can produce bad effects. Feelings of rejection occur if "good" behavior is not recognized. Anger and resentment result if the surgeon uses his role improperly to force compliance with therapy.

Denial

Denial of the actual reality of the situation may occur with an unwillingness to think about the factual nature of the threat or the impending operation. This may be coupled with fantasies which minimize risks and maximize gains to be achieved beyond rational expectations. In such situations fear may be shifted to other aspects of life and unexpected emotional outbursts may occur.

Fear of Narcosis

A specific fear of narcosis may occur. This may cause an aversion to retiring to bed and to sleep, with the production of troublesome insomnia [10-4].

Operation as Punishment

If the impending experience calls up repressed childhood fears, reassurance by those in authority will not effectively alleviate the increased tension. Such fears and tension may arise at times from the interpretation of the impending surgical experience as a punishment for past actions. Guilt feelings may be strong in such cases.

ANTICIPATORY PHASE

It is clear that the preoperative period is of extreme importance in determining the patient's reaction to the actual impact of the operation and to the postoperative response. Janus has studied this anticipatory phase and has described different types of anticipation reactions [10-5].

Moderate Fear Reaction

Most normal and healthy patients experience moderate fear and anxiety. They worry off and on about the impending operative procedure. They are able to see it in a relatively realistic way both as to risk and benefit. They can accept information from the surgeon and other attendants, whether this information is by nature fear-producing or reassuring. Such information is important to the achievement of emotional balance.

The nature of the dangers to be encountered should be clearly explained to the patient. Discussion of methods by which these dangers can be minimized, prevented, or surmounted, is important for reassurance. The protective features of the environment and the attendants must be stressed. It is important that such information be given in terms that patients can understand, and that experiences to be encountered be described as they will be perceived.

Many individuals have had no personal experience with hospitals or operations and need to be informed about events that they will experience both in the hospital setting and in the operating room. Discussions of this type are reassuring to the patient, as they indicate the surgeon's interest and concern. The patient may be reluctant to ask questions about the proposed operation because of the fear of appearing ignorant or because he does not wish to "bother" the authority figure. The surgeon must show his interest by taking time for adequate discussion of any point which is important to the patient.

Preoperative "worry work" is of vital importance to prepare the patient for stress situations and to condition his response. Weiss feels that "the best prevention of an adverse stress reaction is to insure an adequately supported anticipatory phase." [10-6]

High Fear Reaction

In some patients the preoperative period is a time of great fear. This fear may be out of proportion to the realities of the situation in terms of risk and gains, and may be resistant to reassurance by the surgeon. Such people, in general, are neurotic personalities with a high incidence of anxiety reactions. They tend to be excessively nervous and may seek to postpone the operative experience. Such patients seem to be unable to develop adequate emotional strength to prepare themselves for the impending stress. In the intraoperative and postoperative periods these patients remain highly nervous with a lack of confidence and a lack of willingness to accept reassurance from the surgeon.

Low Fear Reaction

A third group of patients may be classified as the low-fear group. These individuals appear outwardly to be extremely calm and to have no preoperative disturbances, such as loss of sleep or inability to work. Such individuals deny the realities of risk or pain and have fantasized no bad effects from the operative experience. They have thus not developed adequate psychic preparation for the impending stress. They may have little difficulty with very minor procedures, but following major procedures where pain and disability may be inevitable, they react with anger and resentment to these discomforts. Since the reality is far worse than the fantasized effect, they tend to blame the surgeon, the staff, and the hospital for the development of pain and discomfort. They may accuse the surgeon of poor treatment, or inattention.

Most of the individuals in this low-fear group are normal, although a few may be neurotic, obsessional, or schizoid. The major problem arises because of lack of an adequate anticipatory phase. Many of these individuals may be shifted from the low-fear group to the moderate or realistic fear group with an important improvement in their ability to withstand the psychologic stress of operation.

Role of the Surgeon

Emotional support seems to be most clearly developed by the production of a trust relationship between the surgeon and the patient [10-7]. This relationship of trust may depend in considerable degree on the past experience of the patient with physicians and surgeons. It is important for the surgeon to empathize with the patient. He must recognize that he is cast in a role of an authority figure, capable, like a parent, of inflicting pleasure or pain. The consistency of the surgeon's relationship with the patient thus becomes extremely important. The patient is abnormally sensitive to signs of annoyance or displeasure, and may overreact if the surgeon fails to fulfill promises of a minor nature, such as delay in the time of a promised hospital visit, or lack of interest in minor discomforts.

The loss of autonomy by the patient and the giving over of life decisions to an authority figure may be well accepted by some patients but poorly accepted or resented by others, depending on past experience. Patients may suffer a feeling of impotence and inferiority progressing in some cases to severe depression, helplessness, and failure to cooperate.

Reassurance and the development of a trust relationship between patient and surgeon is most important for the "high fear reaction" group of patients. The surgeon must be aware of the frequency of temporary

emotional disturbances in this group of patients and develop an em-
pathic understanding of their personality inadequacies.

The surgeon's responsiblity in the "low fear reaction" individuals
is to expose them to reality. This must be done by a realistic discussion
containing fear arousing statements, a sort of rehearsal of crisis. At the
same time such statements must be coupled with reassurance as to the
precautions against danger [10-8].

STRESS IMPACT PHASE

During the actual operative experience and the immediate postoperative days, the specific reactions of the patient as shown in the anticipatory phase will be intensified. If an adequate psychic preparation has
taken place and the personality is strong, the individual can maintain
personality control throughout this phase. All individuals, however,
suffer from feelings of loss of autonomy coupled with worries of isolation (physical abandonment) or rejection (psychological abandonment). Those in attendance on the staff must be clearly aware of the
presence of these fears in all patients, however well concealed. With
high-intensity stress, the patient places more reliance on authority fig-
ures to control the situation. The need for the physical presence of an
attendant, and the need for a sympathetic approach is much greater
under these circumstances. Likewise the lack of such sympathetic attention is more keenly felt [10-9].

POSTIMPACT PHASE

The patient's reaction to the postoperative period will depend in
great measure on the relationship between his expectations and the actual experience. If the expectations have been realistic and the experience is equal to or better than that which was expected, the patient
will relax and become somewhat more self-indulgent. His dependency
becomes somewhat lessened and he is less sensitive to innuendos in the
behavior of the surgeon.

If the anticipation has been unrealistic, and the experience is relatively or actually worse than that expected, negative reactions ensue.
Feelings of victimization increase and rage and grief may be directed
toward those in authority, or inward. A regression to more childlike

behavior may occur. Feelings of impotence increase. Such a patient is very sensitive to actions on the part of those in authority. The patient may resent actions taken without advance warning, and is rebuffed by attitudes which show no acknowledgment of attempts to be "good." Lack of interest in the magnitude of suffering, or lack of attention to protests or pleas for aid and reassurance may be strongly felt. The rage and grief activated by insensitivity on the part of the surgeon and those in attendance may be directed outwardly with overt rage reactions against those in authority, or may be directed inwardly with the development of a feeling of loss of self-esteem and hopelessness.

Isolation

Certain situations may arise that remove the patient from a one-to-one relationship with any authority figure. These occur in some cases due to sensory deprivation, where patients may have eyes closed due to bandaging or edema, hands restrained because of injuries, burns or intravenous lines, speech removed due to the presence of a tracheostomy, and frequent visiting made impossible by isolation techniques. Sensory deprivation produces anxiety, increase in nervous tension, and hallucinations. There is a tendency to rehearsal of memory, meditative thought and reverie, and an increased body awareness [10-10]. These reactions have occurred during studies of sensory deprivation by immersion [10-11], and have been found in patients in a cardiac intensive care unit [10-12]. They also appear to be quite common in patients with severe burns.

In these situations a special effort must be made to provide reassurance and communication to the patient. It is important that an attendant be present whenever possible and that he communicate his presence and his interest in the patient by touch and conversation to prevent intensive feelings of abandonment and rejection. Such feelings become intensified with the passage of time, and patients such as those with severe burns may require constant reassurance and emotional support over many weeks [10-13].

It is very important to involve such patients in active discussion and participation in their own care. Participation reinforces a sense of identity and returns to the patient some measure of control over the situation. Redevelopment of autonomy is important to enable the patient to function in the hospital and at home after discharge.

Role of the Surgeon

The surgeon must understand and accept his central role as the authority figure. It is the surgeon's responsibility to be aware of the frequency of temporary emotional disturbances in surgical patients. He must learn to interpret the patient's reactions in the proper fashion in order to assist the patient in the preoperative anticipatory work of psychic preparation. The patient will be deprived of decision making and will look to the surgeon for the appropriateness and safety of his care. The development of this trust in the patient-doctor relationship is a very significant factor in recovery. Studies of patient reactions have shown the importance of a preoperative visit by such a trusted individual, and of a visit in the recovery room following operation [10-14].

Throughout the hospital course the surgeon must keep clearly in mind the abnormal sensitivity of each patient to feelings of physical and psychological abandonment. His approach to the patient must be gentle, understanding, and patient. This is especially true of patients with chronic or mutilating diseases where constant cheerful reassurance may be difficult to maintain. While caring for such patient, repressed fears of mutilation and death may become strong in the surgeon and in those in attendance on the patient. This may lead them to shun the patient as a reminder of their own mortality. These feelings must be recognized and controlled in order that the staff maintain a continuing supportive role.

RESPONSE OF CHILDREN

Special care must be taken to provide support when infants and children undergo operation. Infants need the presence of a trusted parent [10-2]. The aim is to minimize any disruption of the symbiotic unit and thus to reinforce the baby's sense of security. Normal schedules of sleep and feeding should be maintained whenever possible.

Emotional problems occur most frequently in children aged 1 to 3 years. At this age, the child is sensitive to painful experiences, and is susceptible to the anxiety caused by separation from parents. There has usually been no previous experience with stress situations. Explanations are not understood by children of this age, and they cannot comprehend the reasons for the hospital setting, operating room procedure, or altered daily schedule [10-15].

Postoperatively children in this age group may show negative reactions with disobedience and defiance. They may appear fearful and anxious and may engage in destructive behavior. Such alterations from preoperative behavior probably indicate a feeling of betrayal and loss of trust.

Children in the age group 1–3 appear to be helped most by emotional support in the person of a sympathetic parent, and from understanding attendants. Explanations of needed treatment are important, but seem to be less effective in allaying anxiety [10-16].

Older children can comprehend the purpose of operations more fully, and explanations can help them to develop adequate emtional reserves. Separation anxiety is common in older children also. The latter may view treatment as punishment and careful discussion of benefits to be derived is important. Death fears may be strong in relatively young children and may be associated with anesthesia, intravenous infusions, injections, or restraining apparatus. Sympathetic explanation is frequently needed.

EMOTIONAL PROBLEMS OF THE AGED

Elderly patients vary greatly in emotional stability and in mental acuity. The effects of time, particularly the effects of degenerative vascular disease, are present to some degree in most aged individuals. The addition of the stress of trauma or operation, and the interruption of accustomed activities may produce mental and emotional deterioration. The adverse effects of metabolic, circulatory, and emotional alterations may be cumulative under these circumstances.

Measurable mental deterioration occurs in as many as 25 per cent of surgical patients over 65 years of age (10–17). Many elderly patients easily lose contact with reality when placed in new surroundings. Disorientation and hallucinations may occur at night due to darkness, or after minimal doses of drugs. Depression is common, stemming from a feeling of physical weakness and impotence. Projection of causes of difficulty onto others may lead to paranoid feelings about attendants and family. Immobilization is poorly tolerated, and may accentuate feelings of impotence and/or paranoia.

In the elderly patient hope and interest in life may be extremely important in survival. A reinforcing cycle of responses seems to be at work. Thus some individuals respond to the operative experience with a sense of renewal. They see the procedure as improving their ability to function. They become hopeful and more able to go forward with an increase in ego strength. Other individuals seem mentally depleted. They may question the advisability of the operative procedure and doubt any positive result. Such patients seem less able to go on, and become withdrawn and inactive. This mental state may lead to failure to eat, and failure to thrive, with eventual death.

Although the factors important in determining the response of a patient are not known, certain supportive measures appear valuable. Of utmost importance is the patient's grasp of reality and sense of hope for the future. Whenever possible familiar objects should be near the patient, and frequent visits by close relatives and friends should be encouraged. A strong patient-surgeon relationship is essential. Stress should be placed on discussing a favorable outcome, and on involving the patient as a responsible adult with plans for the future. Return to normal activity should occur as soon as possible.

SPECIAL PROBLEMS

Cardiac Arrest

Patients who have survived a cardiac arrest appear to have intense emotional disturbances not seen in other patients with similar underlying illnesses [10-18]. These reactions may be functional in nature, or may represent varying degrees of brain damage secondary to anoxia. However, the emotional problems of these patients appear to be out of proportion to any organic deficits. Thus it is possible that the disabling nature of these problems may be improved by therapy.

Common findings are insomnia, irritability, and neurotic restriction of activity. Anxiety and fear may be displaced into worry about trivia or projected into worry about relatives or friends. Hallucinations, delusions, and nightmares occur. Discussion of the experience of cardiac arrest, and candid discussion of the patient's fears and anxieties are important before the patient leaves the hospital and establishes new life patterns.

Cardiopulmonary Bypass

Psychiatric omplications appear to be much more frequent in patients after cardiopulmonary bypass than in patients following other types of serious operations. Freyhan and coworkers, after reviewing the postoperative course of 150 patients stated that "no other form of surgery, no matter how severe or psychologically traumatizing, produces psychiatric complications of the reported kind and magnitude." [10-19] Others who have investigated this problem have reported similar findings. Lehmann et al noted psychiatric complications in 15 of 18 patients after bypass and in none of 27 patients after other major surgery [10-20]. Tufo et al found cerebral damage in 20 per cent of patients under 40 years of age, and in 69 per cent of patients over 50 [10-21]. Most authors have related the psychiatric complications to brain damage from perfusion. Both anoxia and microembolism have been implicated.

FATAL ILLNESS

In spite of the many advances in medicine, there are patients who develop incurable diseases and die. The surgeon must play a special role to help such patients. The supportive care that the surgeon can offer depends in great measure on his knowledge of the patient's concept of death and dying, and upon his own background and his own fears of death.

Concept of Death and Dying

Part of the human condition is the inability to conceptualize non-being. Freud said, "In the unconscious everyone of us is convinced of his own immortality." [10-22] This comforting feeling develops early in childhood. Children of 3 or 4 years of age spontaneously develop a denial of death by beliefs in omnipotence, and by some concept of an afterlife [10-23]. This denial or inability to conceptualize death is so strong that it exists even in the face of obvious and imminent life-threatening problems. Norton, in interviewing 25 patients dependent for life on chronic dialysis, indicated that one-half of these patients seemed unable to generalize at all about life and death and were concerned only with the day-to-day activities and details of their dialysis [10-24].

Needs of the Patient

The needs of the patient with a potentially or actually fatal disease seem to be quite clear. He wants to be treated as a living adult person and desires realistic conversation concerning his illness. Most patients want to be told the truth. It must be given to them in such amounts and in such a way that they can understand it and cope with it. Alfred Adler has said, "One should not stab into truth; what may gush out might be destructive." Fatal illness and death is part of life and the patient responds to knowledge of his own condition much as he has responded to other crises throughout his life. He needs sympathetic understanding, and the reassurance that he will have sustained physical and emotional support and will not be abandoned [10-25].

In the initial stages of a fatal illness, the patient is still relatively well and able to live on a satisfactory level. At this time trust in the surgeon must be established by a realistic discussion of the disease and the potentials for treatment. Hope must be sustained even though recovery may be uncommon. At this stage the patient seems more willing to talk about his illness and a great deal of preparation for future trouble may be taken. Enjoyment of life should be encouraged, even with the knowledge of its finite length.

As the disease process advances, the attempt should not be made to produce in the patient a psychotic delusion of improvement. The patient knows that he is getting worse and appreciates confirmation of his own sense of reality from the physician. It is important at this stage that the physician stress the positives in the situation, however. The ability of the patient to breath easily, or the proper function of the intestinal tract become important factors which the patient can see and accept as real things.

In the terminal stages, the patient may show regression to a more childlike state, losing interest in adult matters and becoming more and more dependent on the parental physician figure. The intense fear of the patient in this phase is of abandonment, either physical or psychological. Support must be given by the physician and the staff by visiting the patient often and showing their sympathetic interest by their presence. It has been said that the opposite of love is not hate, it is indifference. Patients may not need the love of each attendant, but above all else they fear indifference. The final moments, very often, see a decrease in sensitivity to surroundings, especially in chronic illness. Sir William Osler commented after witnessing many deaths, "An immense majority die as they were born: oblivious." [10-26]

Reaction of the Surgeon

The sense of omnipotence and immortality on the one hand and the fear of death on the other appear to be stronger in doctors than in other individuals. The physician's experience with death and dying may reinforce this sense of concern about his own mortality. His fear may be somewhat moderated by his knowledge that medication and treatment are available to control pain or discomfort. Thus the physician brings to a patient faced with a fatal illness his personal history and his personal emotional response to the concept of death and dying. In order to care sympathetically and conscientiously for the dying patient the physician must analyze his own feelings. Too many times the physician may fail to face up to his own fears. He may then try to escape the situation by physically abandoning the dying patient or by refusing to discuss with him the problems of death and dying in a realistic way.

A second problem affecting the physician's behavior occurs when a disease is running a fatal course. This is the development of a feeling in the physician that he has "lost" the battle against disease, and therefore he has failed. White has pointed out that "Doctors do not in the long run prevent death." His point is that it is vitally important to cure the patient if that is possible, that that if it is not possible, the physician cannot cease to minister effectively to the patient's needs. He further states, "The physician can succeed when success means that he has tried, he has done his very best, and that his patient has not died alone, has not died unloved, has not died in any more discomfort than necessary." [10-27]

Candid Discussion of Feelings

During the entire course of caring for a patient with a serious or fatal illness, the surgeon must be intensely aware of feelings of anger, resentment, and fear both in the patient and in himself. Patients are angry that they are ill, they are angry that fate has dealt them such a blow. This resentment may be turned toward the physician or the staff, or toward the patient's family. Such feelings should be dicussed with the patient to enable him to verbalize them, and thus relieve the pressure of this undirected anger. The physician's own sense of anger at the patient, of frustration with the patient's reactions, and of frustration with an untreatable illness, should be brought out and discussed with the patient. In this way the patient is being treated as a living adult person who can and should be involved not only in his own attitudes and reactions, but in the attitudes and reactions of those who must remain close to him during his terminal illness [10-28].

Supportive Care

The surgeon's responsibility is much broader and deeper than the treatment of physical illness. He must support the patient in every way possible both as an individual and as a surgeon. Most patients want to be treated as mature, responsible human beings, in a way completely similar to the way they are treated when they are not ill. They want to see the surgeon as a sympathetic, warm, human being, who is trying to help them. They wish to place trust in the surgeon that they will receive the best care and that they will remain of central interest and concern to him as long as they are in his charge. A surgeon, in undertaking the care of another human being, accepts the responsibility to give such supportive care to the best of his ability.

REFERENCES

10-1. Garner, H. H.: Psychiatric aspects of surgery. Indust. Med. Surg. 28:351, 1959.

10-2. Titchener, J. L., and Levine, M.: Surgery as a human experience: the psychodynamics of surgical practice. New York, Oxford Univ. Press, 1960.

10-3. Janis, I. L., and Feshbach, S.: Effects of fear-arousing communications. J. Abnorm. Soc. Psychol. 48:78, 1953.

10-4. Deutsch, H.: Some psychoanalytic observations in surgery. Psychosomat. Med. 4:105, 1942.

10-5. Janis, I. L.: Psychological stress—Psychoanalytic and behavioral studies of surgical patients. New York, Wiley ,1958.

10-6. Weiss, R. J., and Payson, H. E.: Personality disorders; gross stress reaction. In Freedman, A. M., and Kaplan, H. I.: Comprehensive textbook of psychiatry. Baltimore, Williams & Wilkins, 1967, p. 1027.

10-7. Wahl, C. W.: The physician's treatment of the dying patient. Ann. N.Y. Acad. Sci. 164:759, 1969.

10-8. Howland, C., Janis, I. L., and Kelley, H.: Communication and persuasion. New Haven, Yale Univ. Press, 1953.

10-9. Egbert, L. D., Battit, G. E., Turndorf, H., Beecher, H. K.: The Value of the preoperative visit by anesthetist: a study of doctor-patient relationship. JAMA 185:533, 1963.

10-10. Solomon, P.: Sensory deprivation. In Freedman, A. M., and

Kaplan, H. I.: Comprehensive textbook of psychiatry. Baltimore, Williams & Wilkins, 1967, p. 253.

10-11. Lilly, J.: Mental effects of reduction of ordinary levels of physical stimuli on intact healthy persons. Psychiat. Res. Rep. 5:1, 1956.

10-12. Kornfeld, D. S., Zimberg, S., Malm, J. R.: Psychiatric complications of open heart surgery. New Engl. J. Med. 273:287, 1965.

10-13. Andersen, N. J. C., Noyes, R., Jr., Hartford, C. E., Brodland, G., and Proctor, S.: Management of emotional reactions in seriously burned adults. New Engl. J. Med. 286:65, 1972.

10-14. Winkelstein, C., Blacher, R. S., and Meyer, B. C.: Psychiatric observation on surgical patients in recovery room. N.Y. State J. Med. 65:865, 1965.

10-15. Levy, D. M.: Psychic trauma of operations in children. Am. J. Dis. Child. 69:7, 1945.

10-16. Prugh, D. G., Staub, E. M., Sands, H. H., Kirschbaum, R. M., and Lenihan, E. A.: A study of the emotional reactions of children and families to hospitalization and illness. Am. J. Orthopsychiat. 23:70, 1953.

10-17. Titchener, J., Zwerling, I., Gottshalk, L., Levine, M.: Psychological reactions of the aged in surgery. Am. Arch. Neurol. Psychiat. 79:63, 1958.

10-18. Druss, R. G., and Kornfeld, D. S.: The survivors of cardiac arrest. JAMA 201:291, 1967.

10-19. Freyhan, F. A., Gianelli, S., O'Connell, R. A., and Mayo, J. A.: Psychiatric complications following open-heart surgery. Comprehensive Psychiat. 12:181, 1971.

10-20. Lehmann, H. J., Grahmann, H., Hauss, K., Rodewald, G. W., Schmitz, T. Akute organische Psychosyndrome nach Herzoperationen. Nervenartz 39:529, 1968.

10-21. Tufo, H. M., Ostfeld, A. M., Shekelle, R.: Central neurvous system dysfunction following open-heart surgery. JAMA 212:1333, 1970.

10-22. Freud, S.: Thoughts for the times on war and death. London, Hogarth Press, 1915, 1957.

10-23. Rochlin, G.: Griefs and discontents. Boston, Little Brown, 1965.

10-24. Norton, C. E.: Attitudes toward living and dying in patients on chronic hemodyialysis. Ann. N.Y. Acad. Sci. 164:720, 1969.

10-25. Krant, M. J.: The organized care of the dying patient. Hosp. Pract. 7:101, 1972.

10-26. MacDermott, H. E.: Notes on the early editions of Osler's textbook of medicine. Ann. Med. Hist. 6:224, 1934.

10-27. White, L. P.: The self-image of the physician and the care of dying patients. Ann. N.Y. Acad. Sci. 164:822, 1969.

10-28. Senescu, R.: The problem of establishing communication with the seriously ill patient. Ann. N.Y. Acad. Sci. 164:699, 1969.

INDEX

The numbers within brackets in boldface type identify references to the literature pertaining to the subjects indexed. The references are found at the end of each chapter; the first digit of each hyphenated number is the chapter number.

259